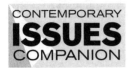

Women's Health

Other Books of Related Interest:

Opposing Viewpoints Series

Abortion

America in the Twenty-First Century

Eating Disorders

Health

Health Care

Mental Illness

Obesity

Teenage Pregnancy

At Issue Series

Anorexia

Antidepressants

Bulimia

Cosmetic Surgery

Reproductive Technology

Should Abortion Rights Be Restricted?

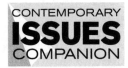

Women's Health

Christina Fisanick, Book Editor

GREENHAVEN PRESS

An imprint of Thomson Gale, a part of The Thomson Corporation

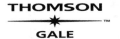

Detroit • New York • San Francisco • San Diego • New Haven, Conn.
Waterville, Maine • London • Munich

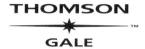

Bonnie Szumski, *Publisher*
Helen Cothran, *Managing Editor*
David M. Haugen, *Series Editor*

© 2006 Thomson Gale, a part of The Thomson Corporation.

Thomson and Star logo are trademarks and Gale and Greenhaven Press are registered trademarks used herein under license.

For more information, contact:
Greenhaven Press
27500 Drake Rd.
Farmington Hills, MI 48331-3535
Or you can visit our Internet site at http://www.gale.com

LIBRARY OF CONGRESS CATALOGING-IN-PUBLICATION DATA

Women's Health / Christina Fisanick, book editor
    p. cm. -- (Contemporary issues companion)
    Includes bibliographical references and index.
    0-7377-2468-4 (lib. : alk. paper) 0-7377-2469-2 (pbk. : alk. paper)
    1. Women--Health and hygiene. I. Fisanick, Christina. II. Series.
    RA564.85.W66653 2006
    613'.04244--dc22
                                                                2005058941

Printed in the United States of America
10 9 8 7 6 5 4 3 2 1

Contents

Foreword

In the news, on the streets, and in neighborhoods, individuals are confronted with a variety of social problems. Such problems may affect people directly: A young woman may struggle with depression, suspect a friend of having bulimia, or watch a loved one battle cancer. And even the issues that do not directly affect her private life—such as religious cults, domestic violence, or legalized gambling—still impact the larger society in which she lives. Discovering and analyzing the complexities of issues that encompass communal and societal realms as well as the world of personal experience is a valuable educational goal in the modern world.

Effectively addressing social problems requires familiarity with a constantly changing stream of data. Becoming well informed about today's controversies is an intricate process that often involves reading myriad primary and secondary sources, analyzing political debates, weighing various experts' opinions—even listening to firsthand accounts of those directly affected by the issue. For students and general observers, this can be a daunting task because of the sheer volume of information available in books, periodicals, on the evening news, and on the Internet. Researching the consequences of legalized gambling, for example, might entail sifting through congressional testimony on gambling's societal effects, examining private studies on Indian gaming, perusing numerous Web sites devoted to Internet betting, and reading essays written by lottery winners as well as interviews with recovering compulsive gamblers. Obtaining valuable information can be time-consuming—since it often requires researchers to pore over numerous documents and commentaries before discovering a source relevant to their particular investigation.

Greenhaven's Contemporary Issues Companion series seeks to assist this process of research by providing readers with useful and pertinent information about today's complex issues. Each volume in this anthology series focuses on a topic of current interest, presenting informative and thought-provoking selections written from a wide variety of viewpoints. The readings selected by the editors include such diverse sources as personal accounts and case studies, pertinent factual and statistical articles, and relevant commentaries and overviews. This diversity of sources and views, found in every Contemporary Issues Companion, offers readers a broad perspective in one convenient volume.

In addition, each title in the Contemporary Issues Companion series is designed especially for young adults. The selections included in every volume are chosen for their accessibility and are expertly edited in consideration of both the reading and comprehension levels of the audience. The structure of the anthologies also enhances accessibility. An introductory essay places each issue in context and provides helpful facts such as historical background or current statistics and legislation that pertain to the topic. The chapters that follow organize the material and focus on specific aspects of the book's topic. Every essay is introduced by a brief summary of its main points and biographical information about the author. These summaries aid in comprehension and can also serve to direct readers to material of immediate interest and need. Finally, a comprehensive index allows readers to efficiently scan and locate content.

The Contemporary Issues Companion series is an ideal launching point for research on a particular topic. Each anthology in the series is composed of readings taken from an extensive gamut of resources, including periodicals, newspapers, books, government documents, the publications of private and public organizations, and Internet Web sites. In these volumes, readers will find factual support suitable for use in reports, debates, speeches, and research papers. The anthologies also facilitate further research, featuring a book and periodical bibliography and a list of organizations to contact for additional information.

A perfect resource for both students and the general reader, Greenhaven's Contemporary Issues Companion series is sure to be a valued source of current, readable information on social problems that interest young adults. It is the editors' hope that readers will find the Contemporary Issues Companion series useful as a starting point to formulate their own opinions about and answers to the complex issues of the present day.

Introduction

Throughout much of the history of westernized medicine, women's health concerns have been largely ignored. For centuries, medicine was practiced by men with men in mind. Therefore, medical knowledge of how the human body works was built upon a male model. While there are certain similarities between male and female bodies, large differences exist between the two, and those differences can radically alter the ways in which physicians diagnose and treat men's and women's health problems. In addition, the lack of understanding of women's unique health concerns has traditionally meant that they do not receive the attention they deserve. There is, perhaps, no better example of this negligence than the case of breast cancer.

Breast cancer impacts thousands of women each year and remains a leading cause of death for American women. However, as many women's health advocates attest, breast cancer has historically been mistreated and has received less research and funding than male-centered cancers, such as prostate cancer. Although women's health initiatives since the 1970s have done much to spread awareness and raise money for research, advocates say that federal and state support for breast cancer research and prevention needs much improvement. According to Breast Cancer Action, a grassroots organization of breast cancer survivors and their supporters, "While breast cancer issues continue to attract the interest of legislators, meaningful action at both the state and federal levels remains elusive." Therefore, even though the medical community has begun to take the disease seriously, without the support of government agencies, progress toward a cure will remain slow, and breast cancer will continue taking women's lives.

Written records from as far back as ancient Egypt and Greece indicate that breast cancer has long confused women and their physicians. While writings reveal that a variety of treatments were used, from the application of topical ointments to the surgical removal of the breast, none of these early records points to a cure. Centuries later, a cure has still to be discovered. Today, women are more likely to survive breast cancer, but the odds are not as favorable as most women would hope, given the survival and cure rate of other cancers such as testicular and skin cancer.

According to the National Cancer Institute, 13.2 percent of American women will be diagnosed with breast cancer in their lifetimes. Although earlier detection and better treatments have shown a slight decrease in the number of deaths from breast cancer since the early 1990s, the American Cancer Society estimates that about 1 in 33 American women will die from breast cancer (40,410 women in 2005 alone). Women's health care advocates argue that these numbers remain high because not enough money and effort has been spent on breast cancer research and awareness. Shahla Masood, professor and associate chair of the Department of Pathology at the University of Florida Health Science Center and chief of pathology and laboratory medicine at the University Medical Center, urges that "The government, state legislators, community leaders and the public should be effectively educated to understand the ultimate lifesaving and cost-saving effects of research."

Up until the early twentieth century, there was little advancement in the treatment of breast cancer. In the 1920s surgeon William Halsted popularized the radical mastectomy as the main course of treatment. This standard practice, which involved the removal of the affected breast, lymph nodes, and frequently, part of the rib cage, remained commonplace until the 1970s. While research conducted in the 1980s and 1990s would reveal that radical mastectomies may not have saved as many lives as once expected, it seemed to physicians in Halstead's time to be the only means to rescue women from cancer's deadly effects. For women patients, the problem with the procedure was that it not only disfigured their bodies, but it was often done without their input. The decision to perform a radical mastectomy was made on the operating table. Women expecting exploratory surgery for a chest ailment would wake up to find one or both of their breasts removed if the surgeon discovered a cancerous tumor. While women endured this method of treatment for decades, the women's movement would dramatically change the way breast cancer patients were treated.

In the early 1970s women's health advocacy became a strong political movement, and women began to realize the importance of taking a larger role in all aspects of their lives, especially their health. Breast cancer quickly became the leading cause for women's health groups because women believed that not enough was being done to educate, diagnose, and cure women with the disease. Although the groundwork for breast cancer advocacy began in the 1950s with the formation of the American Cancer Society's Reach to Recovery program, which joined women who had had mastectomies with women who had just been diagnosed with the disease, breast cancer largely remained a silent issue. No one talked about it publicly, in part because the female breast was a highly sexualized symbol in American culture. In addition, it was difficult for women to speak up when dealing with their doctors because, prior to the women's movement, physicians were seen as paternalistic authority figures and were not supposed to be questioned. In an interview aired on National Public Radio, Barron H. Lerner, author of *The Breast Cancer Wars*, characterizes the male-centered practice of medicine in the 1950s and 1960s:

> Doctors at that time really didn't want to hear women questioning what they were going to do. They didn't want women to go see other doctors and get second opinions and the state of affairs as it was enabled them in essence to silence women patients. They weren't doing this because they were

horrible people, but male doctors were used to running the show and they didn't like women interfering with the way things were occurring.

All of that changed in the 1970s with the advent of the women's health advocacy movement. Women felt empowered to speak up about the way their health care was being managed. To raise public awareness about the particular health needs of women and to help women play an active role in their own health care, women's health organizations were formed. One such organization, the Boston Women's Health Book Collective, published the influential book *Our Bodies, Ourselves* in 1970. It was one of the first studies written by women with the goal of providing accurate, timely information about women's health issues. *Our Bodies, Ourselves* inspired the work of countless women's health advocates including those women who would later become strong voices for women's breast health.

Like today's campaign to raise awareness about women and heart disease, the women fighting for breast cancer awareness in the early 1970s were greatly aided by famous people who spoke up about the disease. In 1972 former child actress turned politician, Shirley Temple Black, was diagnosed with breast cancer and was the first celebrity to go public with the disease. She did so to encourage other women to get tested. Soon after, other well-known women publicly announced that they had breast cancer, including first lady Betty Ford. The efforts of women's health advocacy groups and celebrity spokeswomen worked at increasing early detection. According to breast cancer researcher Susan Love, author of *Dr. Susan Love's Breast Book*, following these public pronouncements "there was a dramatic increase in the number of women in America who got mammograms, and the number of breast cancer cases diagnosed."

These early women's health efforts spawned a generation of breast cancer advocacy groups that would go on to fight for more and better breast cancer research, to raise public awareness about the seriousness of the disease, and to encourage women to take an active role in their health by teaching them to perform monthly breast exams and to get regular mammograms. One such organization, The Susan G. Komen Breast Cancer Foundation, has been the most public force of breast cancer advocacy in the United States since its formation in 1983. It continues to lead national and international campaigns to raise awareness about the disease and regularly sponsors the Race for the Cure marathon and other fund-raising events. However, despite all of the attention it has received since the 1970s, including the nationally recognized pink ribbons that decorate everything from cars to purses to energy bar wrappers, there remains no cure for breast cancer.

The breast cancer advocacy movement laid the groundwork for future women's health campaigns, including the campaign to raise awareness about women's heart disease. Born out of a need to take action and to become more involved with their bodies and health care decisions, breast cancer advocates pushed the disease into the public eye and have helped thousands of women seek early detection and treatment for the disease. Subsequent generations of breast cancer advocates face a long, tough road that will likely include fighting insurance companies for more access to mammograms and other early detection procedures, battling with industries whose environmental pollutants increase the risks of breast cancer, and continuing to encourage women to take an active role in their own health care. Certainly the biggest challenge that the next generation of breast cancer advocates face is to increase funding for breast cancer research and treatment from government agencies. Although much of the gender bias involving breast cancer diagnosis and treatment has been dissolved by the efforts of breast cancer advocates, until government agencies begin to take the illness seriously by allocating funding and legislation for better research and treatment, the disease will continue to claim the lives of numerous victims.

Women's health dominates the lists of concerns for many women's organizations around the world. *Contemporary Issues Companion: Women's Health* helps illuminate some of the most important issues impacting women's health. By presenting essays, reports, and personal narratives, this volume attempts to bring attention to many issues that affect women's health, including women and weight, women and reproduction, women and mental illness, and international women's health issues.

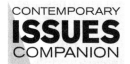

CHAPTER 1

The Impact of Culture on Women's Health

American Culture Exalts an Unnatural and Dangerous Female Body Image

Frances M. Berg

Many American women feel dissatisfied with the way their bodies look, which often prompts them to seek dangerous means of weight loss. These include starvation dieting, diet drugs, and other methods that can lead to disordered eating and serious health problems. In this excerpt from Women Afraid to Eat: Breaking Free in Today's Weight-Obsessed World, *Frances M. Berg, internationally known authority on weight and eating, points to the media, advertising, and societal views about women for such distorted views of body image. She argues that these elements begin to impact girls as young as age two. She concludes that disordered body image is a major health risk for women and that it spawns from society's desire to control women in the public and private sectors. In addition to* Women Afraid to Eat, *Berg has authored eight other books. She is a licensed nutritionist, a family wellness specialist, and an adjunct professor at the University of North Dakota School of Medicine.*

At no time in history have women been so pressured to be thin. Thinness is sold on every street corner, and the wonderful diversity of women, their inner beauty and well-being, is rejected. Women—even those of below average weight—look at themselves and see a body that is too big or is oversized in one part or another.

Our culture is deeply ambivalent about women and their bodies.

"Women are idealized and denigrated, protected and abused, encouraged and discriminated against. By the time

Frances M. Berg, *Women Afraid to Eat: Breaking Free in Today's Weight-Obsessed World*. Hettinger, ND: Healthy Weight Network, 2001. Copyright © 2001 by Frances M. Berg. All rights reserved. Reproduced by permission.

most girls become women, they have confused and conflicting feelings about their place in the world. This confusion manifests itself in a dissatisfaction with their bodies and their appearance. Before long, their confused and conflicting feelings boil down to one issue: Fat," write Jane Hirschmann and Carol Munter in *When Women Stop Hating Their Bodies*.

Perhaps in decades to come, our culture will place less importance on the "ideal female body"—the term should be an obscenity—and women can feel good about themselves in their natural sizes and shapes.

But not now.

The Distorted Media Mirror

Page through almost any magazine, look at almost every television show. Notice anything about the women there?

It seems as if there is literally one model—one who is thin, youthful, beautiful and who, in reality, represents perhaps five percent of women in America.

Where are the other 95 percent? We need to be seeing women in a wider range of shapes, sizes, ages, and attractiveness on television, in advertising, magazines, and the movies. We need lots more role models for the 95 percent of girls and young women who will never achieve that "ideal look"— which of course is often reshaped through plastic surgery, or retouched, airbrushed, and computer-enhanced on the page.

But how can we expect girls and women to know what a normal, healthy body looks like when all they see are the victims of starvation being praised and glorified for their skeletal structures?

Women on television seem to get thinner each year. Their fashionable faces are now gaunt and hollow-cheeked, reflected everywhere in real life. It hurts to see a lineup of thin girls from the side—high school cheerleaders, for instance—their stomachs caved in, bony clavicles and hip bones protruding. Where are the bodies they have worked so hard to perfect?

There's no body. Only bones, arms, legs, hair and that frightening skeletal face, screaming out cheers—or maybe, screaming for help from a society that has abandoned them.

Media—in all its forms—is a powerful messenger. . . .

The two institutions of the "ideal woman"—the Miss America Pageant and Playboy—are being represented by women who are thinner and thinner every year and proportionately smaller in the hips, as a 30-year survey vividly illustrates. Now the typical contestant or model weighs in at 13 to 19 percent below expected weight, and has almost no curve at the hip. The clinical criteria for anorexia nervosa is 15 percent below expected weight.

"Pathologically underweight women are being held up as cultural ideals," laments Dr. David Greenfeld, medical director of the Yale-New Haven Hospital Adolescent and Young Adult Treatment Unit.

This distorted picture of reality portrayed through the media adversely affects girls and women in three ways, says Karin Jasper, PhD, of the Women's Center Toronto.

The distortions include:

1. Frequently propagating myths and falsehoods
2. Normalizing or even glamorizing what is abnormal or unhealthy
3. Creating the false impression that all women are alike by failing to represent whole segments of the real world

These false messages contribute to the confusion of women, thinness obsession, and prevalence of eating disorders, says Jasper.

Women and girls believe them, respond to them. . . .

The Power of Advertising

But who has the power to resist the bombardment?

Advertising expertly conveys the message that "you're not okay—and here's what you need to buy to fix what's wrong."

Advertising sells body dissatisfaction a thousand times a day to women and men who are being set up by the constant stream of gaunt images in the media. The perfect model guarantees our desire to fix our "ugly fat" or other "ugly" features through buying product X.

We buy the product; it doesn't work. We're left with dissatisfaction about a feature we hadn't even noticed before, and the belief that there is one more thing wrong with us. Then we go out and buy more.

It's a wildly successful strategy.

Advertising is a $130 billion industry and the most powerful educational force in America. It has designed the cultural ideals of the last two or three decades.

Media pressure to be thin is stronger now than at any time in the last 19 years. A recent study found that television diet promotions, nonexistent in 1973, now comprise about five percent of TV advertisements.

Jean Kilbourne, EdD, author of *Still Killing Us Softly: Advertising and the Obsession with Thinness*, argues that advertising overpowers almost every other cultural message through sheer force. The average American sees 1,500 ads per day and spends a year and a half of a lifetime watching TV commercials.

"The tyranny of the ideal image makes almost all of us feel inferior," Kilbourne says. "We are taught to hate our bodies, and thus learn to hate ourselves. This self-hatred takes an enormous toll . . . (in) feelings of inferiority, anxiety, insecurity, and depression."

The thinness craze is lucrative for the fashion and tobacco industry; for the makers of body products, weight loss products and services, diet drinks, and for every industry from trucks to whiskey that advertises with striking models posed with the product.

Advertisers are "killing us softly," warns Kilbourne. Yet she says they will never voluntarily change, because it is "profitable for women to feel terrible about themselves.". . .

Dieting Never Ends

Pressures to be thin are especially acute on college campuses today. Food restriction is taking its toll as young women struggle to attain an emaciated ideal.

"Instead of being strong and creative and full of resilience, so many young women I speak to on college campuses, again the best and the brightest, are barely making it through at a level of survival," warns Naomi Wolf. "Because they're exhausted. And they're exhausted because they're starving or vomiting compulsively. This generation's voice is diminished, their reasoning powers are blunted. And this is America's future leadership."

But the passion for thinness is by no means confined to younger women—a phase they pass through, and then outgrow as they mature. In today's world women of all ages are threatened by body dissatisfaction, and older women are not exempt.

Studies show that even after age 70, a great many women are still dieting. Among women over age 60 who are not overweight, more than 22 percent are trying to lose weight, according to national statistics from the Centers of Disease Control. This includes nearly 25 percent of Mexican American women, 22.4 percent of white women, and 14.4 percent of African American women—all of them within normal weight range. . . .

Socializing Young Girls

Where does it all start? By age 2, girls are watching television and starting their daily exposure to messages that show successful women are thin. They are hearing their mothers, teachers, older sisters, and women in general objectify, distrust, and battle their bodies in order to make them acceptably thin. They are hearing their fathers, brothers, and important males in their lives talk about and judge women's bodies.

As preschoolers, they learn that certain types of foods will make them fat. Six-year-olds know eating fat is bad, and that people who are fat should diet and exercise. More seriously, a substantial number of girls in primary grades are so concerned about their bodies, they have already tried to lose weight. Weight preoccupation and body dissatisfaction are occurring earlier and earlier. By fourth grade, 40 percent or more of girls "diet" at least occasionally. Those who do not are gathering information and forming values and opinions.

Modern culture is youth-centered, yet in many ways it does not provide an environment that is nurturing or supportive for the healthy growth and development of girls. In fact, it nurtures serious problems.

"A girl-poisoning culture . . . a girl-destroying place," psychologist Mary Pipher brands our society in her book, *Reviving Ophelia.*

Pipher says that in early adolescence girls are expected to sacrifice the parts of themselves that our culture considers masculine on the altar of social acceptability. They have to shrink their souls down to petite size.

With nearly all the messages about thinness aimed at girls and women, some researchers see strong ties between the American public health crisis over weight and eating disorders and an intentional cultural oppression of women. The attack messages work best when the target is young. And young adolescent girls are most vulnerable.

"I am deeply concerned about what is happening to young girls in our society today," says Paula Levine, PhD, former president of Eating Disorders Awareness and Prevention. "Young girls up until the age of 11 are confident, unafraid of conflict, and willing to say exactly what is on their minds. As they enter puberty, however, they adjust to society's messages about what young women are 'supposed' to be—nice, kind, caring, self-sacrificing, agreeable and compliant." . . .

Is It About Women's Freedom?

What kind of culture would require its women to remain hungry and half-nourished?

The answer, some would say, is a culture that has given women more freedom than it is comfortable with.

Is this, then, about women's freedom? That's one explanation.

In this view, women entering the marketplace in such large numbers threaten the power of corporate and political institutions, as well as threatening male power. Keeping women physically small, immature, semi-starved, and diverted from life's real issues diminishes their power as competent individuals, and reduces their chances of building strong careers.

This travesty is not being perpetuated on women by individual men, for the most part—men, after all, have female friends, lovers, wives, sisters, daughters they care about—but by the political power structure and multinational corporations bent on shaping women into the ultimate consumers, perennially dissatisfied with their appearance.

From a feminist perspective, the selling of thinness and the ignoring of the diversity of real women is seen as a manipulative tool to prevent women from gaining power in the work force. The adverse effects of self starvation in the ceaseless quest for a thin body keeps women passive, preoccupied, dependent, and off track from career ambitions. It keeps them in their place as objects to be viewed or pleasured, or used as recreational toys or playmates.

Obsessed with Dieting and Thinness

Dieting and thinness came to be female preoccupations when women got the right to vote around 1920. Never before had there been idealized "the look of sickness, the look of poverty, and the look of nervous exhaustion." The new, leaner form re-placed the more curvaceous one with startling rapidity, Wolf says, in a great weight shift that must be understood as one of the major historical developments of the century, a direct so-lution to the threat posed by the women's movement and their newly-won economic and reproductive freedom.

"Prolonged and periodic caloric restriction is a means to take the teeth out of this revolution . . . so that women just reaching for power would become weak, preoccupied, and mentally ill in useful ways and in astonishing proportions," says Wolf.

The cultural fixation on female thinness is not about beauty but female obedience, Wolf charges. It's "about how much social freedom women are going to get away with."

The "good girl" today is a thin girl, one who keeps her ap-petite for food (and for power, sex and equality) under con-trol, agrees Kilbourne. Girls are still being admonished to keep their place, to not compete too seriously.

Control Over Women

Both men and women are conditioned and socialized to feel that women must be controlled, kept in their place. Women, of course, internalize these messages, says Kilbourne. "Ironi-cally, what is considered sexy today is a look that almost to-tally suppresses female secondary sexual characteristics, such as large breasts and hips. Thinness is related to decreased fer-tility and sexuality in women."

Kilbourne argues that women are allowed success in the workplace if they focus on being thin, maintain a fragile, waifish image, and do not take up too much space. "The pur-suit of thinness is a way to compete without threatening men."

Another explanation for the idealization of the lean boyish female figure is that as women have moved into previously male-dominated activities, the traditional feminine shape has developed negative connotations, while the masculine shape symbolizes self-discipline and competency. Thus the rejection of the maternal body can be seen as women's revolt against the sometimes impossible demands of trying to fill both career and reproductive roles.

Kilbourne warns, "This is not a trivial issue; it cuts to the very heart of women's energy, power and self-esteem. This is a major public health problem, one that endangers the lives of young girls and women."

Gender Biases Negatively Impact Women's Health Care Worldwide

Piroska Östlin, Asha George, and Gita Sen

A major worldwide health gap exists between women and men. In the following selection, Piroska Östlin, Asha George, and Gita Sen discuss the global impact of such gender biases. For example, in countries where social discrimination against women is pervasive, women's life expectancy is below that of men. In addition, in developing countries maternal mortality rates are high and indicate a much more disturbing problem with health equality in these countries. Part of the problem, according to the authors, is that many health care systems either do not recognize the health care needs specific to women or simply focus on reproductive health alone. Furthermore, some health care systems do not treat female patients with the same amount of respect as male patients. Complicating these problems is the lack of clinical research on drugs and treatments that take women's unique biology into consideration. The authors argue that while there have been some recent examples of improvement of women's access to health care, there is much that needs to be done to reduce gender bias around the world. Östlin, George, and Sen conduct research on women's global health care issues and their work has appeared in a number of books, including Health and Social Justice: Politics, Ideology, and Inequity in the Distribution of Disease, *from which this selection is taken.*

In many health care systems there is often insufficient attention to the differential needs of men and women in planning health services. As a result, health services for women often focus on only reproductive functions. The widespread priority of maternal child health has focused primarily on children to the relative neglect of the mothers. Important women's health issues, unrelated to their reproductive role, tend to be shortchanged. In Tanzania, the gender bias in adolescent health policies has led to a disproportionate focus on female reproductive health to the virtual exclusion of policies addressing both male adolescents and young women with nonreproductive health needs.

Gender inequality may also be manifest in the ways men and women are treated by the health care system. Mounting evidence suggests that male and female health providers may be gender biased in their perception of patient preferences and problems. Patient-physician differences in age, class, sex, race, or ethnicity are found to accentuate gender bias in quality of care. Studies from rural communities in West Africa and from Chile have shown that women are not always treated with respect by health providers. In many societies women complain about lack of privacy, confidentiality, and information about treatment options. Underpaid, overworked, and gender-insensitive health care workers will be unlikely to communicate with, examine, and prescribe appropriately for women (or men). Not surprisingly, women in some cultures prefer traditional providers (healers), who take the time to listen and explain ailments in easily understood terms. Given that many women are reluctant to be examined by male doctors, the lack of female medical personnel—itself a reflection of gender bias in educational opportunity—is an important barrier to utilization for many women.

Studies in the Netherlands, Sweden, and the United States highlight gender inequalities in the provision of certain technologies or treatment services for the same disease. Women with heart disease are less likely than men to receive coronary bypass surgery, and women are less likely to receive organ transplants such as kidney transplants. In the case of lung cancer, it has been found that women are less likely than men to have cytological tests of sputum ordered by their doctors.

A wide variety of sociodemographic factors such as employment status and age interact with gender relations to generate inequalities in accessing health care. Although health care services may be available, girls and women may be unable to access them due to discrimination within the household, granting preferential allocation of resources to male needs. Girls are likely to receive less expensive and more home-based care than boys and also more likely to suffer from outright neglect of their health needs than boys. In general, vulnerable sections of society, such as poor, illiterate, or less educated rural women, may not even be aware of their legal rights to adequate health care.

Clinical Research

Medical research and clinical trials for new drugs have been heavily criticized during the last decade for their general lack of a gender perspective. Health problems that specifically or predominantly affect women have received less attention and funding than research on health problems mainly prevalent among men. The lack of research is obvious in areas concerning menstruation and nonlethal chronic diseases that affect women disproportionately, such as rheumatism, fibromyalgia, and chronic fatigue syndrome. The only exception to this trend is contraceptive research, which has historically neglected male methods and focused on controlling fertility rather than on enhancing women's contraceptive and reproductive options.

In the field of occupational health and safety, women are overlooked in toxicological studies. Even when women are considered, their biological specificity is seldom noted. For example, the effects of occupational exposures on lactating women have received little study despite research results indicating the adverse health effects of their exposure to certain chemicals. This is a particularly important issue for women, as their greater level of body fat means that they store more fat-soluble toxic material even when exposed to the same levels as men.

An even more serious problem has been the exclusion of female subjects from study populations for medical and drug research. One rationale for excluding female subjects from research is that the menstrual cycle introduces a potentially confounding variable. Additional grounds for omitting women of childbearing age is the fear that experimental treatments or drugs may affect their fertility. Experimental use of treatment might, moreover, expose fetuses to unknown risk. Despite such concerns, the consequences for women of interpreting research results based on studies of male models and without convincing evidence of their applicability to women, continue to be harmful to women. Accumulating evidence shows that technology for diagnoses, treatment of diseases, and rehabilitation programs are not adapted to the specific characteristics and needs of women in general, let alone to women in various socioeconomic circumstances or cultural backgrounds.

Encouragingly, emerging research on gender differences in cardiovascular epidemiology has revealed the serious shortcomings of applying "male-based" diagnostic techniques and treatments to female patients. In part, this stems from increased recognition that symptoms of heart attack differ significantly between men and women. Of particular concern is recent evidence that life-threatening delays in diagnosis (via EKG) of women may occur because of lack of awareness of the unique nature of female symptomatology. . . .

Lack of Access to Medical Services

Many developing countries continue to suffer from weak or deteriorating health services, infrastructures, and unaffordable services, a situation that disproportionately affects women. The inadequacy and lack of affordability of health services are compounded by physical and psychological barriers to care. At the national level, there have been some attempts to tackle the cost and affordability barriers to health services for women. For example, both South Africa and Sri Lanka provide free maternal and infant health services. Flat fee structures that cover not only regular antenatal and postnatal care but also delivery care, including complications, may be one way to ensure that cost barriers do not prevent families from bringing women in for such services, especially during obstetric emergencies. When health insurance schemes are introduced, care should be taken to ensure that poor women are adequately covered.

Even such services as are available or affordable to the poor in general may still be out of the reach for girls and women. In some settings, this is a matter of distance or transport access, which may make it impossible for girls or women to visit health centers, particularly where gender taboos limit women's mobility. Upgrading local (village-level) health centers, setting up systems for reliable emergency transport, and making it possible for women and their attendants to stay near a health facility can help to bridge this gap. Such measures have yielded good results in countries such as Cuba, Sri Lanka, Uganda, and, in the Matlab project, in Bangladesh. . . .

Particularly nefarious are the health systems that exacerbate health inequalities through lack of gender sensitivity. All too often health policy makers tend to view women primarily as "reproducers" and narrowly focus their attention on women in the reproductive ages. In 1994, the International Conference on Population and Development attempted to correct this bias by including actions to meet the health needs of girls, adolescents, and older women.

Positive Examples

Perhaps the most comprehensive attempt to design a more holistic policy has been the Comprehensive Program for

Women's Health Care, which was created in Brazil in 1983. This program includes a range of reproductive and sexual health services, as well as occupational and mental health services. It includes not only women in the reproductive ages but also postmenopausal women and preadolescents, and it emphasizes that women need access to both preventive and curative care as well as information about their bodies and health.

Another positive example of an integrated and gender-sensitive health policy is the "Health for Women, Women for Health" policy enunciated by the Ministry of Health in Colombia in 1992, which explicitly aims to reduce gender inequalities through a comprehensive approach. Its five programs include the promotion of self-help, reproductive health and sexuality, violence prevention and care for victims of violence, mental health, and occupational health. The policy document states explicitly that a "woman has the right to treatment and care from the health services as a whole being, with specific needs—according to her age, activity, social class, race, and place of origin, and not to be treated exclusively as a biological reproducer. She has the right to respectful and dignified treatment by health workers of her body, her fears, and her needs for intimacy and privacy."

Thus, quality of care and attention to women's health needs throughout the life cycle are critical components in the health system—and as essential to ensuring utilization as physical access and affordability.

Reducing Gender Bias

Promoting gender equality and equity also requires tackling gender biases in communities and households through community education, empowering women, and training boys and men to reduce gender biases by promoting gender-sensitive behavior and reducing violence. The International Conference on Population and Development initiated a broad-based policy discussion on this subject. There are also many examples from both developed and developing countries of person-based strategies aimed at strengthening individuals in disadvantaged positions. From a gender equity perspective, such strategies have focused mainly on strengthening women to better respond to, and control determinants of, health in the physical or social environment. The most effective interventions have been those with an *empowerment* focus. They aim to help disadvantaged women to gain their rights, improve their access to essential facilities and services, address perceived deficiencies in their knowledge, acquire personal or social skills, and thereby improve their health.

Empowerment initiatives aim at encouraging both sexes to challenge gender stereotypes. One of these projects, described by Craft, is The Girl Child Project, established by the Family Planning Association of Pakistan. The project raises awareness among young girls and their families about unfair and unnecessary discrimination against girls and thereby promotes the status and the value of the girl child. For example, according to the girls involved, the project made them aware that unequal food allocation in the family is wrong. In fact, just a few years ago, Pakistan was one of the countries where the female life expectancy was inferior to male life expectancy. By 1997, this situation had reversed, indicating a positive trend toward the greater gender equity in longevity.

In Bangladesh, one of the initiatives (BRAC) integrated into a poverty alleviation project focused on the empowerment of poor rural women by provision of women's microcredit and female education. Gender equity in health was improved considerably via increased economic independence and improved social status relative to men in both public and personal spheres. Positive changes were also reported in food allocation and educational attainment that led to decreasing male bias in a society where preference for sons is deeply rooted. The BRAC initiative, designed to increase gender equity, has also successfully contributed to the sharp decline in the socioeconomic gap in child mortality but has not significantly altered the gender gap in child mortality.

Obesity Is a Major Health Threat to Women

Tori Hudson

Studies estimate that as many as 50 percent of Americans are overweight or obese and that up to 40 percent of American women are trying to lose weight at any given time, prompting national health care advisers to consider obesity an epidemic. According to Tori Hudson, professor of gynecology at the National College of Naturopathic Medicine in Portland, Oregon, and author of the Women's Encyclopedia of Natural Medicine, *the health risks for women who are overweight or obese are severe. She points to studies that demonstrate that women with a body mass index (BMI) above twenty-seven are at high risk for developing diabetes, high blood pressure, high cholesterol, and osteoarthritis. Hudson also discusses the health benefits of weight loss, including a reduction in cholesterol levels, high blood pressure, certain cancers, and sleep disorders.*

Obesity is characterized by an excess of body fat and is a serious and pervasive health problem in America today, particularly among women. The prevalence of overweight in women is defined as a body mass index (BMI) of 25 to 29.9 and obesity as a BMI equal to or greater than 30.

Your BMI is an objective scientific measure that uses your height and weight. You can calculate your BMI by dividing your weight in kilograms by the square of your height in meters. In other words BMI = $Kg/[(m).sup.2]$. One variable BMI fails to consider is lean body mass. It is possible for a healthy, muscular individual with very low body fat to be classified obese using the BMI formula.

Tori Hudson, "Obesity in Women—Women's Health Update," *Townsend Letter for Doctors and Patients,* August/September 2002. Copyright © 2002 by *Townsend Letter for Doctors and Patients.* All rights reserved. Reproduced by permission.

1 inch = 2.54 cm 1 meter = 100 cm 1 lb = 0.45359237 Kg

More than half of American women and men are overweight or obese. Although about 9% more men than women between the ages of 20 and 80 have a BMI of 25 or greater, more women than men are seriously overweight, qualifying as obese, having a BMI of 30 or greater. 25% of US women and 19.5% of men are obese with higher percentages for minority women, (36.7% non-Hispanic African American women and 33.3% Mexican American women). The prevalence of Caucasian women who are overweight or obese, ranges from 18% among 25 to 34 year olds to 35% among 55 to 64 year olds. Sixty percent of African American women aged 45 to 65 are either overweight or obese.

The incidence of obesity is increasing in America at a disturbing and alarming rate. Since 1980, obesity in both men and women has increased by over 50%. It is estimated that 33% to 40% of American women are trying to lose weight at any given time, as well as 20% to 24% of the men.

Health Consequences

Issues of overweight or obesity should be viewed as a medical problem with significant excess morbidity and mortality. A feminist philosophical defense of overweight, a sort of "fat and proud" political position, may have value in changing cultural views of beauty and the ideal woman as thin, and even underweight, but both attitudes are harmful to the psychological and physical well-being of women.

Most research shows that health risks are lowest in individuals with a BMI between 19 and 25. Health risks start to significantly increase when the BMI exceeds 27. At this point, nutritional and lifestyle strategies should be implemented. Once the BMI exceeds 30, more effective rigorous interventions should be initiated.

In addition to BMI, waist-to-hip ratios are also an important measurement. Overweight women and those with the "apple" fat distribution are at greater risk for developing coronary artery disease than are slim women and those with the "pear" fat pattern. This abdominal obesity also increases the risk of high blood pressure and diabetes and may lower the HDL-cholesterol level and raise the triglyceride level. A desirable ratio of waist-to-hip for middle-age women is <0.8. The abdomen is measured at the largest point, and divided by the hip measurement. This is called the waist-hip ratio.

Overweight and obesity are linked to numerous health risks and consequences. Increasing weight is associated with increased mortality. As the percentage of weight increases, mortality increases. Women who have the lowest mortality in the US are women who weigh at least 15% less than the average weight for other women her age.

Overweight women are three times more likely to have high blood pressure than women who are not overweight. Even individuals who are only 20% overweight have an eight-fold increase in the incidence of hypertension over those of normal weight. Obesity is an established risk factor for hypertension and dyslipidemia as well as cardiac morbidity and mortality. The Nurses' Health Study of over 115,000 women also found a strong correlation between body weight and mortality. Hyperlipidemia is 1.5 times greater in overweight individuals than in lean people. In addition, high-density lipoprotein (HDL) cholesterol is lower in obese people and elevated triglyceride levels have also been associated with weight gain.

The association of obesity with insulin resistance and hyperinsulinemia is increasingly understood as both cause and effect. Insulin resistance and hyperinsulinemia leads to the development of type 2 diabetes. Much of our information on the interplay of DM II and obesity in women comes from the Nurses' Health Study. Researchers found that even women with a BMI within the range of what is usually considered to be normal (23 to 23.9) had a 3.5 times greater risk of developing type 2 diabetes than women with a BMI less than 22. They also found that the risk more steeply rises after the BMI exceeds 27. Women with a BMI equal or greater than 35 had 58.2 times greater age-adjusted risk than those with a BMI less than 22. Onset of type 2 diabetes during pregnancy occurs much more frequently in pregnant obese women and one such review indicated at least a quadrupled risk increase.

Hypertension, hyperlipidemia, cardiovascular disease and diabetes are the best known consequences of obesity. However, overweight and obesity are associated with significant health consequences from other causes as well. Several cancers are associated with obesity—gallbladder, breast, cervix, uterus and ovaries. The risk of gallbladder disease increases with weight to the point that 28% to 45% of morbidly obese individuals have gallbladder disease.

Obesity is also a risk factor for osteoarthritis, particularly of the knee, hip and back. In women, weight is the single most important known risk factor for the development of osteoarthritis.

Anovulation and infertility are also associated with an increased BMI. A BMI of 28 to 29.9 was associated with a 2.4 fold risk of infertility compared with a BMI of 20 to 21.9.

As many as one third of obese patients who seek medical treatment for their weight also engage in episodes of binge eating. This then is associated with more severe obesity and frequent cycling of weight. Underlying psychological disorders or histories are important to explore with obese individuals. Adult survivors of sexual abuse, current or recent sexual abuse, abusive relationships and depression are often masked or dealt with by overeating and subsequent weight problems. On the other hand, obesity itself can lead to depression, anxiety, low self-esteem and body image and social withdrawal.

Health Benefits of Weight Loss

Weight loss is a fundamental and necessary intervention in people who are overweight and obese with cardiac risk factors. Even modest weight loss can have significant impact on cardiovascular disease risk factors. Only a 5% to 10% weight loss has been shown to improve triglycerides, total cholesterol, and reduce blood pressure in hypertensive individuals. Weight loss has also been shown to reduce blood pressure in those with high-normal blood pressure in addition to preventing hypertension. Weight loss has been shown to produce a direct linear reduction in blood pressure. For each kilogram of weight lost, systolic blood pressure was reduced by 0.43 mm Hg and diastolic blood pressure by 0.33 mm Hg.

Weight loss should be considered a priority treatment for type 2 diabetes and the related metabolic disorders. Again, as is true with hypertension and abnormal lipid profiles, a weight loss of only 10% can improve blood sugar control in diabetics who are obese. Even modest weight loss reduces the risk of type 2 diabetes-related mortality. In a US study of Caucasian women, researchers found that a weight loss of 1 to 19 lbs resulted in a 44% reduction in mortality related to diabetes. More significant weight loss of 20 lbs was surprisingly related to a lesser reduction in mortality, only 33%.

Weight loss can also reduce mortality from obesity-related cancers such as gallbladder, breast, cervix, uterus and ovaries. A weight loss of 1 to 19 lbs was associated with a 53% reduction in mortality from these obesity-related cancers. More than 20 lbs was associated with a 39% reduction.

Small amounts of weight loss can improve sleep apnea in people who are mildly to moderately obese. A weight loss of 11 lbs. in people who have a BMI of 25 or greater can reduce their risk of developing osteoarthritis by more than 50%.

Last but not least, losing weight can produce many psychological benefits. Improvements in feelings about their bodies, self-esteem and depression can be significant. Although prejudice and discrimination are a shameful fact of life faced by obese people in our culture, weight loss offers freedom from these consequences.

Approaches to Weight Loss

Overweight and obesity should be treated as a chronic disease. It requires long term attention to nutrition, exercise and activity patterns, other lifestyle issues and exploration of personal/psychological issues. Some individuals may benefit from nutritional or herbal supplementation and others might need to consider medication.

Weight loss efforts should be individualized and directed toward a slow but steady weight loss. Generally, weight loss should not exceed 1 to 1.5 lb per week. Most overweight people will not be able to achieve an ideal body weight. Rather than try to achieve ideal weight, the goal should be the best weight for health benefits.

Overweight Women Suffer
Abuse in Silence

Susan Koppelman

*Many American women feel ashamed of how their bodies look,
writes Susan Koppelman. Pressured by the media, which exclusively promotes the thin female form, some girls and women develop loathing for their bodies over time. According to Koppelman, this body hatred is multiplied several times over for
overweight girls who are often teased and abused by other children and even adults, which can lead to feelings of shame and
worthlessness. As a young girl grows into adulthood, she carries
these negative feelings with her. Koppelman argues that overweight women are also targets of physical, mental, and sexual
abuse thereby continuing the cycle begun in childhood. She further states that because overweight women have learned to accept themselves as worthless, they often suffer these abuses in silence. She finds hope, however, in recent efforts to recognize the
plight of overweight women in American culture. Koppelman is
the editor of multiple anthologies of women's short stories and is
considered a foremost expert on women's short fiction.*

Criticism of a girl or woman's body by those whom she
trusts most, with whom she is most intimate, and to
whom she is most vulnerable is not only one of many ways
girls and women are abused, it is one of the most common.
As Dorothy Taber, a rehabilitation counselor working with
persons with psychological and physiological disabilities, has
commented, "Over the many years that I have worked as a
counselor of women, every female client I have worked with
over a period of time, of months, regarding partner abuse, has
commented about the trauma caused by negative remarks

Susan Koppelman, "Fat Women and Abuse," *Off Our Backs*, vol. 34, November/
December 2004. Copyright © 2004 by Off Our Backs, Inc. Reproduced by permission.

concerning their body by their abusers, adding to the basic shame that most women apparently have about their bodies. One would expect for persons with disfiguring conditions to have negative bodily images. But this isn't necessarily so. Many people with average, healthy, 'normal,' and often beautiful physicality believe they are ugly, homely, and misshapen." The criticism can be couched in any number of ways, and whether it is presented "lovingly" as "for your own good" or brutally as "you deserve to be punished for what you have done to yourself" or "what you have become," it is always painful for the fat woman to experience and it *never* feels like love. Whether the words come from a husband, a domestic partner, a lover, a parent, a sibling, or a friend, they always wound.

The Roots of Abuse

The earlier the criticism begins in the life of a person, the more permanent and long-term the damage can be. And when the criticism begins after or in conjunction with some highly stressful event (and a stressful event can be a welcome event, such as pregnancy or child-birth as well as a catastrophe, such as illness or the loss of a loved one), the person being criticized is even more vulnerable than at other times. Wounding remarks about a person's natural appearance delivered by those who are supposed to love you are toxic. Being told you are too anything—too fat, too thin, too tall, too short, underdeveloped, over-developed, too dark—not only is a blow to one's self-esteem and one's natural sense of being at one with one's own body, but it undermines one's ability to trust in the safety of anyone's love.

In heterosexual marriages, abusive husbands frequently try to control their wives' appearances as if their wives were pieces of furniture, possessed by the men and vulnerable to reupholstering. It isn't clear whether the men are really dissatisfied with their wives' bodies at a personal level or if they are just desperate to have their wives conform to current beauty ideals because their wives' appearances reflect on them. No doubt the men couldn't make the distinction between their own personal preferences and their career ambitions themselves.

Fat Girls and Abuse

Fat girls often experience emotional and sometimes physical abuse, bullying, intimidation, and humiliation from their peers in public settings such as school or playgrounds. There is seldom interference in this bullying by adults for all the reasons that we know: adults rarely interfere in the torturing of children by each other. Perhaps the most significant reason they don't interfere in the case of fat children is their conviction that the abuse is deserved.

The catalogue of abusive behaviors by parents of many fat girls and fat young women is increasingly familiar to children as the unwarranted hysteria about the so-called "obesity epidemic" reaches truly pandemic proportions. Children perceived to have "too much body" are put through a common routine of shaming, blaming, depriving, and distancing by parents with means and determination to govern the bodies of their fat youngsters for their own good: Children as young as three months are put on diets. Food restriction and withholding is a common memory for adults who grew up as fat children. Children whose parents have means are sent to "fat camps" that are run like institutions designed to punish; some are even sent to twelve-month "fat schools" to be schooled in self-hatred, self-deprivation, and self-surrender.

Our society has a general penchant for abusing the powerless and the weak and punishing the different; it makes perfect sense that people with fat bodies will be abused. And, since appearances are markers of such significance in determining social value in our culture, it makes perfect sense that abusers will attack those bodies in every way possible, including physically, sexually, verbally, medically, and financially.

In fact, it often doesn't matter if a woman is really fat; if she lives in a fat-fearing, fat-hating culture and she is in an intimate relationship with an abuser, she will be told, scolded for, punished because she is fat. Even if she isn't. This abuse is perhaps only the most literal expression of the punishment our culture imposes on bodies that dare to transgress from the socially prescribed norms.

In the world at large, the abuse of fat women and girls remains a secret, surrounded by fear, shame, and self-blame. And, like abused women in general, many fat women are likely to go on suffering in silence unless and until the larger truths are told, and blame is placed where it belongs—on the abusers, and on the culture that produces them.

Fat Acceptance Movement

Although heterosexual women, and men, both fat men and those men called "fat admirers," have participated in the founding, development, and maintenance of the fat acceptance movement on many fronts, the most radical literature about fat oppression and fat liberation has come from the lesbian feminist fat liberation movement. The literature of fat liberation (or size acceptance, or the fat civil rights movement) is a bravura literature ranging in tenor from pugnacious to lyrical, ironic to heartbroken, furious to comical. It includes the genres anticipated in such a literature: moving memoirs, heartbreaking confessions, declarations of love and alliance for those like the writer, white-jawed rants, murderous tirades, well-reasoned arguments, angry manifestos, three point sermons—and poetry that reflects all of these sentiments and more. As a body of literature, it is relatively new, seeming to begin with writing by the Fat Liberation Underground in 1974.

After these early publications, there has been a steadily increasing river of books and articles and periodicals addressing women and fatness. That more and more of these publications were feminist and represent something truly new in literature, that is, the voice of the fat woman herself, the fat woman as agent rather than object, is a consequence of many factors.

During these three decades [since 1974], fat people have begun to find our authentic literary voices and used them to portray and protest our outsider role in society, to question the science used to condemn us, and to assert our determination to define ourselves and live on our own terms. During the same period of years, eating disorders, including anorexia, bulimia, exercise addiction, binge eating, and compulsive overeating, seem to occur with greater frequency and the attention focused on these conditions has increased.

Whether a woman is a radical fat liberationist, fat, proud, defiant, and bound and determined to claim her rightful share of joy, to have her say, to take up space on the dance floors of life, to look you in the eye and say, Fat! So? or a size acceptance advocate who believes passionately in the all-rightness, the normalcy, the beauty of women of all shapes and sizes, or a woman who is still in hiding, still wearing that black raincoat in summer, who hasn't been swimming in decades, who spends her days and nights waiting for her life to begin once she "does something about herself"—all of these women are telling their stories, writing poems and essays and manifestos and novels and short stories that say, "this is how it is for ME!"

I am grateful for their stories.

Female Genital Mutilation Can Be a Safe Cultural Rite of Passage

Richard A. Shweder

Female genital mutilation (FGM), or the intentional cutting and removal of the clitoris or vaginal lips, is an age-old ritual that is part of the cultural practices in a number of African countries and other countries around the world. Since this ritual has been brought to the attention of women all over the world, women's rights and human rights groups have stepped forward to declare it barbaric and violent, damaging the physical, mental, and sexual health of the young girls who undergo the procedure. In the following excerpt Richard A. Shweder takes a closer look at FGM and attempts to sort out the truths behind the practice. Ultimately, Shweder argues that FGM can be a safe procedure that is not demoralizing to girls and women. In fact, he asserts, women within cultures who practice FGM often desire to have the procedure performed. He believes that cultural differences have blinded many anti-FGM activists and have resulted in discriminatory views about the practice. Shweder is a writer and educator who has lived and taught in Africa.

Coming-of-age ceremonies and gender-identity ceremonies involving genital alterations are embraced by, and deeply embedded in the lives of, many African women, not only in Africa but in Europe and the United States as well. Estimates of the number of contemporary African women who participate in these practices vary widely and wildly between eighty million and two hundred million. In general, these women keep their secrets secret. They have not been inclined to ex-

Richard A. Shweder, "What About 'Female Genital Mutilation'? And Why Understanding Culture Matters in the First Place," *Daedalus*, vol. 129, Fall 2000. Copyright © 2000 by the American Academy of Arts and Sciences. Reproduced by permission of the Russell Sage Foundation.

pose the most intimate parts of their bodies to public examination and they have not been in the habit of making their case on the op-ed pages of American newspapers, in the halls of Congress, or at academic meetings. So it was an extraordinary event to witness Fuambai Ahmadu, an initiate and an anthropologist, stand up and state that the oft-repeated claims "regarding adverse effects [of female circumcision] on women's sexuality do not tally with the experiences of most Kono women," including her own. Ahmadu was twenty-two years old and sexually experienced when she returned to Sierra Leone to be circumcised, so at least in her own case she knows what she is talking about. Most Kono women uphold the practice of female (and male) circumcision and positively evaluate its consequences for their psychological, social, spiritual, and physical well-being. Ahmadu went on to suggest that Kono girls and women feel empowered by the initiation ceremony and she described some of the reasons why. . . .

In the social and intellectual circles in which most Americans travel it has been so "politically correct" to deplore female circumcision that the alarming claims and representations of anti-"FGM" advocacy groups (images of African parents routinely and for hundreds of years disfiguring, maiming, and murdering their female children and depriving them of their capacity for a sexual response) have not been carefully scrutinized with regard to reliable evidence. Nor have they been cross-examined by freethinking minds through a process of systematic rebuttal. Quite the contrary; the facts on the ground and the correct moral attitude for "good guys" have been taken to be so self-evident that merely posing the rhetorical question "what about FGM?" is presumed to function as an obvious counterargument to cultural pluralism and to define a clear limit to any feelings of tolerance for alternative ways of life. This is unfortunate, because in this case there is good reason to believe that the case is far less onesided than supposed, that the "bad guys" are not really all that bad, that the values of pluralism should be upheld, and that the "good guys" may have rushed to judgment and gotten an awful lot rather wrong. . . .

Moral Pluralism and the "Mutual Yuck Response"

People recoil at each other's practices and say "yuck" at each other all over the world. When it comes to female genital alterations, however, the "mutual yuck" response is particularly intense and may even approach a sense of mutual outrage or horror. From a purely descriptive point of view, that particular type of modification of the "natural" body is routine and normal in many ethnic groups. For example, national prevalence rates of 80–98 percent have been reported for Egypt, Ethiopia, the Gambia, Mali, Sierra Leone, Somalia, and the Sudan. In African nations where the overall prevalence rate is lower—for example, 50 percent in Kenya, 43 percent in Cote d'Ivoire, 30 percent in Ghana—this is typically because some ethnic groups in those countries have a tradition of female circumcision while other ethnic groups do not. For example, within Ghana the ethnic groups in the north and the east circumcise girls (and boys), while the ethnic groups in the south have no tradition of female circumcision. In general, for both boys and girls the best predictor of circumcision (versus the absence of it) is ethnicity or cultural group affiliation. For example, circumcision is customary for the Kono of Sierra Leone, but for the Wolof of Senegal it is not. For women within these groups, one key factor—their cultural affiliation—trumps other predictors of behavior, such as educational level or socioeconomic status. Among the Kono, even women with a secondary-school or college education are circumcised, while Senegalese Wolof women—including the illiterate and unschooled—are not.

Native Views on FGM

There are other notable facts about this cultural practice. For one thing, most African women do not think about circumcision in human-rights terms. Women who endorse female circumcision typically argue that it is an important part of their cultural heritage or their religion, while women who do not endorse the practice typically argue that it is not permitted by their cultural heritage or their religion.

Second, among members of ethnic groups for whom female circumcision is part of their cultural heritage approval ratings for the custom are generally rather high. According to the Sudan Demographic and Health Survey of 1989–1990, which was conducted in northern and central Sudan, out of 3,805 women interviewed 89 percent were circumcised. Of the women who were circumcised, 96 percent said they had circumcised or would circumcise their daughters. When asked whether they favored continuation of the practice, 90 percent of circumcised women said they favored its continuation. . . .

Third, although ethnic group affiliation is the best predictor of who circumcises and who does not, the timing and form of the operation are not consistent across groups. Thus, there is enormous variability in the age at which the surgery is normally performed (any time from birth to the late teenage years). There is also enormous variability in the traditional style and degree of surgery (from a cut in the prepuce covering the clitoris to the complete "smoothing out" of the genital area by removing all visible parts of the clitoris and most if not all of the labia). In some ethnic groups (for example, in Somalia and the Sudan) the "smoothing out" operation is concluded by stitching closed the vaginal opening, with the aim of enhancing fertility and protecting the womb. The latter procedure, often referred to as "infibulation" or Pharaonic circumcision, is not typical in most circumcising ethnic groups, although it has received a good deal of attention in the anti-

"FGM" literature. It is estimated that it occurs in about 15 percent of all African cases.

In places where the practice of female circumcision is popular, including Somalia and the Sudan, it is widely believed by women that these genital alterations improve their bodies and make them more beautiful, more feminine, more civilized, more honorable. . . .

As hard as it may be for "us" to believe, in places where female circumcision is commonplace it is not only popular but fashionable. As hard as it may be for "us" to believe (and I recognize that for some of "us" this is really hard to believe), many women in places such as Mali, Somalia, Egypt, Kenya, and Chad are repulsed by the idea of unmodified female genitals. They view unmodified genitals as ugly, unrefined, and undignified, and hence not fully human. They associate unmodified genitals with life outside of or at the bottom of civilized society. "Yuck," they think to themselves; "what kind of barbarians are these who don't circumcise their genitals?"

Cultural Views on FGM

The "yuck" is, of course, mutual. Female genital alterations are not routine and normal for members of mainstream or majority populations in Europe, the United States, China, Japan, and other parts of the world, including South Africa. For members of those cultures the very thought of female genital surgery produces an unpleasant visceral reaction; although it should be noted that for many of us the detailed visualization of any kind of surgery—a bypass operation, an abortion, a sex change operation, a breast implantation, a face lift, or even a decorative eyebrow or tongue piercing—produces an unpleasant visceral reaction. In other words, merely contemplating a surgery, especially on the face or the genitals, can be quite upsetting or revolting, even when the surgery seems fully justified from our own "native point of view."

In the United States and Europe the practice of genital surgery has been disparaged as "mutilation." It has been re-described as rape or torture and associated with the night-mare of some brutal patriarchal male (or perhaps a Victorian gynecologist) grabbing a young woman or girl, pulling her into the back room screaming and kicking, and using a knife or razor blade to deprive her of her sexuality. Various dra-matic and disturbing claims have been made about the health hazards and harmful side effects of African genital operations, including the loss of a capacity to experience sexual pleasure.

Saying "yuck" to the practice has become a symbol of op-position to the oppression of women and of one's support for their emancipation around the world. Eliminating the practice has become a high-priority mission for many Western femi-nists (and for some human-rights activists in Africa, who, un-derstandably enough, often, although not invariably, come from noncircumcising ethnic groups) and for some interna-tional health and human-rights organizations (for example, the World Health Organization, Amnesty International, and Equality Now).

Outside of Africa, especially in the United States and Eu-rope, opposition to female circumcision has become so "po-litically correct" that until very recently most anti-anti-"FGM" criticism has been defensive, superficial, or sympathetic. The sympathetic criticisms are mainly critiques of counterproduc-tive "eradication" tactics. They provide advice on how to be more effective as an anti-"FGM" activist. . . .

In general, the purported facts about female circumcision go unquestioned, the moral implications of the case are thought to be obvious, and the mere query "what about FGM?" is presumed to function in and of itself as a knock-down argument against both cultural pluralism and any incli-nation toward tolerance.

So What about FGM?

So what about "FGM"? I shall treat this as a real question deserving a considered response rather than as a rhetorical query intended to terminate all debate. For starters, the practice of genital alteration is a rather poor example of gender inequality or of society picking on women. Surveying the world, one finds very few cultures, if any, in which genital surgeries are performed on girls but not boys, although there are many cultures in which they are performed only on boys or on both sexes. The male genital alterations often take place in adolescence and they can involve major modifications (including sub-incision, in which the penis is split along the line of the urethra). Considering the prevalence, timing, and intensity of the relevant initiation rites, and viewing genital alteration on a worldwide scale, one is hard pressed to argue that it is an obvious instance of a gender inequity disfavoring girls. Quite the contrary; social recognition of the ritual transformation of both boys and girls into a more mature status as empowered men and women is not infrequently a major point of the ceremony. In other words, female circumcision, when and where it occurs in Africa, is much more a case of society treating boys and girls equally before the common law and inducting them into responsible adulthood in parallel ways. . . .

In those cases of female genital alteration with which I am most familiar (I have lived and taught in Kenya, where the practice is routine for some ethnic groups), the adolescent girls who undergo the ritual initiation look forward to it. It is an ordeal and it can be painful (especially if done "naturally" without anesthesia), but it is viewed as a test of courage. It is an event organized and controlled by women, who have their own view of the aesthetics of the body—a different view from ours about what is civilized, dignified, and beautiful. The girl's parents are not trying to be cruel to their daughter—African parents love their children too. No one is raped or tortured. There is a celebration surrounding the event.

What about the devastating negative effects on health and sexuality that are vividly portrayed in the anti-"FGM" literature? When it comes to hard-nosed scientific investigations of the consequences of female genital surgeries on sexuality and health, there are relatively few methodologically sound studies. As [Carla] Obermeyer [a medical anthropologist and epidemiologist from Harvard University] discovered in her medical review, most of the published literature is "data-free" or else relies on sensational testimonials, secondhand reports, or inadequate samples. Judged against basic epidemiological research standards, much of the published empirical evidence, including some of the most widely cited publications in the anti-"FGM" advocacy literature (including the influential Hosken Report), are fatally flawed. Nevertheless, there is some science worth considering in thinking about female circumcision, which leads Obermeyer to conclude that the global discourse about the health and sexual consequences of the practice is not sufficiently supplied with credible evidence. . . .

In other words, the alarmist claims that are a standard feature of the anti-"FGM" advocacy literature that African traditions of circumcision have "maimed or killed untold numbers of women and girls" and deprived them of their sexuality may not be true. Given the most reliable, even if limited, scientific evidence at hand, those claims should be viewed with skepticism and not accepted as fact, no matter how many times they are uncritically recapitulated on the editorial pages of the New York Times or poignantly invoked in a journalistic essay on PBS. . . .

The real facts, I would suggest, are quite otherwise. With regard to the consequences of genital surgeries, the weight of the evidence suggests that the overwhelming majority of youthful female initiates in countries such as Mali, Kenya, and Sierra Leone believe they have been improved (physically, socially, and spiritually) by the ceremonial ordeal and symbolic process (including the pain) associated with initiation. The evidence indicates that most of these youthful initiates manage to be (in their own estimation) "improved" without disastrous or even major short-term or long-term consequences for their health. . . .

This is not to say that we should not worry about the documented 4–16 percent urinary infection rate associated with these surgeries, or the 7–13 percent of cases in which there is excessive bleeding, or the 1 percent rate of septicemia. . . . What I do want to suggest, however, is that the current sense of shock, horror, and righteous "Western" indignation directed against the mothers of Mali, Somalia, Egypt, Sierra Leone, Ethiopia, the Gambia, and the Sudan is misguided, and rather disturbingly misinformed. . . .

FGM is Not an Open-and-Shut Case

Imagine an African mother living in the United States who holds the following convictions. She believes that her daughters as well as her sons should be able to improve their looks and their marriage prospects, enter into a covenant with God, and be honored as adult members of the community via circumcision. Imagine that her proposed surgical procedure (for example, a cut in the prepuce that covers the clitoris) is no more substantial from a medical point of view than the customary American male circumcision operation. Why should we not extend that option to the Kono parents of daughters as well as to the Jewish parents of sons, for example? Principles of gender equity, due process before the law, religious and cultural freedom, and family privacy would seem to support the option. . . .

I have also suggested that merely posing the question "What about FGM?" is not an argument against cultural pluralism. With accurate scientific information and sufficient cultural understanding it is possible to see the (not unreasonable) point of such practices for those for whom they are meaningful. Seeing the cultural point and getting the scientific facts straight is where tolerance begins. Our cherished ideals of tolerance (including the ideal of being "pro-choice") would not amount to very much if all they amounted to was our willingness to eat each other's foods and to grant each other permission to enter different houses of worship for a couple of hours on the weekend. Tolerance means setting aside our readily aroused and powerfully negative feelings about the practices of immigrant minority groups long enough to get the facts straight and engage the "other" in a serious moral dialogue. It should take far more than overheated rhetoric and offended sensibilities to justify a cultural "eradication" campaign. Needless to say, the question of tolerance versus eradication of other peoples' valued ways of life is not just a women's issue.

The controversy over female circumcision in Africa is not an open-and-shut case. Given the high stakes involved, I believe it is a responsibility of cultural pluralists—both men and women—who are knowledgeable about African circumcision practices to step forward, speak out, and educate the public about this practice. There are many African women who, out of a sense of modesty, privacy, loyalty, or a well-founded sense of fear, may hesitate to speak for themselves. And it is a responsibility of everyone, anti-"FGM" activists and cultural pluralists alike, to insist on evenhandedness and the highest standards of reason and evidence in any public policy debate on this topic—or at least to insist that there is a public policy debate, with all sides and voices fully represented.

Female Genital Mutilation Causes Severe Health Problems

Loretta M. Kopelman

Female genital cutting or circumcision, which is commonly prac-ticed in Africa, India, and other developing countries, is consid-ered a form of mutilation and abuse in many industrialized na-tions. Global health organizations, including the International Federation of Gynecology and Obstetrics and the World Health Organization, also condemn the practice saying that it violates human rights and leads to mental and physical health problems. Although women and men from countries where the procedure is commonly performed continue to support the practice, a world-wide outcry has been issued in hopes of eliminating the proce-dure. In the following selection Loretta M. Kopelman approaches the subject of female genital mutilation (FGM) from ethical and medical standpoints. She refers to the continued support for and the practice of FGM as relying on a kind of ethical relativism, which states that people from one culture have no right to judge what occurs in another. She argues that global human rights su-persede the rights of one nation or community. In addition, Ko-pelman explains the many possible health complications of FGM, including complications that are immediate, such as pain, bleed-ing, and tetanus, and complications that are long-term, such as urinary tract infections, chronic pelvic infections, and dangerous labor and delivery. She concludes that the only way to stop this practice is through education and activism. Kopelman is a pro-

Loretta M. Kopelman, "Female Genital Circumcision and Conventionalist Ethical Rela-tivism," *Globalizing Feminist Bioethics: Crosscultural Perspectives*, edited by Rose-marie Tong, with Gwen Anderson and Aida Santos. New York: Westview Press, 2001. Copyright © 2001 by Westview Press, a member of the Perseus Books Group. Repro-duced by permission.

fessor in the Department of Medical Humanities at the Brody School of Medicine at East Carolina University and is the founding president of the American Society for Bioethics in the Humanities.

In many parts of the world female genital cutting, child marriages, and denying girls the same opportunities for schooling that boys receive are regarded as violations of the law. Female genital cutting . . . is viewed as mutilation and abuse in many parts of the world, including the United Kingdom, France, Canada, and the United States. National medical societies such as the American Medical Association and influential international agencies including UNICEF, the International Federation of Gynecology and Obstetrics, and the World Health Organization (WHO) openly condemn and try to stop these practices. Around the world, women's groups protest the practice of female genital cutting and infibulation, denying that it is just a cultural issue and arguing that these rites should be treated with the same vigor as other human rights violations.

Defining the Practice

These procedures involve the removal of some, or all, of the external female genitalia, denying women orgasms and causing disease, disability, and death in women, girls, and infants in these regions. These surgical rites, usually performed on girls between infancy and puberty, are intended to promote chastity, religion, group identity, cleanliness, health, family values, and marriage. Most of the people practicing this ritual are Muslim, but it is neither required by the Koran nor practiced in the spiritual center of Islam, Saudi Arabia. These rites predate the introduction of Islam into these regions.

At least 80 million living women have had some form of this mutilation, and each year 4–5 million girls have it done. It is hard to collect data, however, since these rites are technically illegal in many of these countries, the unenforced remnants of colonial days. . . .

The Center for Disease Control estimates that around 48,000 girls currently living in the United States are likely to undergo these rites, over half of them living in the New York City area. Parents sometimes believe it is especially important to have these procedures done in the United States, since they view it as a sex-obsessed society where it is especially necessary to control female sexuality. . . . These parents fear they will lose control of their daughters if they go uncircumcised. Immigrants generally get around laws prohibiting these rites by taking their girls back home or going to practitioners within their communities. . . .

Ethical Relativism

Female genital cutting or circumcision is commonly classified according to three types. Type 1 circumcision is the removal of the clitoral hood or prepuce (skin around the clitoris). Type 2, or intermediary circumcision, is the removal of the entire clitoris and most or all of the labia minora. Type 3, or pharaonic circumcision, is the removal of the clitoris, labia minora, and parts of the labia majora. Infibulation refers to stitching shut the wound to the vulva from genital cutting, leaving a tiny opening so that the woman can pass urine and menstrual flow.

People who want to continue these practices resent cross-cultural criticisms, seeing them as assaults on their social traditions and identity. A version of ethical relativism supports their judgment, holding that people from other cultures have no legitimate basis for such condemnation. [Author] Anthony Flew defines ethical relativism as follows: "To be a relativist about values is to maintain that there are no universal standards of good and bad, right and wrong." To avoid confusion with other definitions of "ethical relativism," I will, following [scholar] Louis P. Pojam, call this position *conventionalist ethi-*

cal relativism. It denies the existence of any underlying universal moral principles among cultures, asserting that moral principles depend entirely on cultural notions and acceptances. It rejects all forms of objectivism (a view that social differences can have underlying similarities with universal validity). [Philosopher] David Hume disavowed conventionalist ethical relativism when he wrote, "Many of the forms of breeding are arbitrary and casual; but the thing expressed by them is still the same. A Spaniard goes out of his own house before his guest, to signify that he leaves him master of all. In other countries, the landlord walks out last, as a common mark of deference and regard." . . .

Female genital cutting and infibulation serve as a test case for conventionalist ethical relativism because these rites have widespread approval within the cultures that practice them and thus on this theory are right. Yet they have widespread disapproval outside their cultures for reasons that seem compelling but on this theory lack any moral authority. Thus many discussions in ethics about female genital mutilation examine which forms of ethical relativism entail that genital cutting is a justifiable practice in societies that approve it. . . .

Morbidity and Mortality of Female Genital Circumcision

Of the three forms of female genital mutilation, Type 1 is the least mutilating and, unlike the other types, may not preclude orgasm. Type 1 circumcision, however, is very difficult to perform without removing additional tissue. Types 2 and 3 are the most popular forms of circumcision and preclude orgasms. These rituals are so widespread that they probably contribute to the belief of men and woman in these regions that sex cannot be pleasurable for women, other than knowing that they bring pleasure to their husbands. More than three-quarters of the girls in the Sudan, Somalia, Ethiopia, Egypt, and other north African and southern Arabian countries undergo type 2 or type 3 circumcision, with many of the others circumcised by type 1. One survey by [Asthma] El Dareer [(1982)] shows that over 98 percent of Sudanese women have had this ritual surgery, 12 percent with type 2 and 83 percent with type 3.

A series of pioneering studies conducted in the Sudan by El Dareer, in Sierra Leone by [Olayinka] Koso-Thomas [(1987)], and in Somalia by [Ruquiya H.D.] Abdalla [(1982)] document that female genital cutting harms girls and women in many ways, having both short- and long-term complications. Later studies confirmed their findings. The operation causes immediate problems that can even be fatal. They find initial problems are pain, bleeding, infection, tetanus, and shock. The degree of harm correlates with the type of circumcision. El Dareer found that bleeding occurred in all forms of circumcision, accounting for 21.3 percent of the immediate medical problems; infections are frequent because the surgical conditions are often unhygienic. She also found that the inability to pass urine was common, constituting 21.7 percent of the immediate complications. Finally, she found that these rites cause many long-term medical complications, including difficulty in the consummation of marriage and hazardous labor and delivery. Of the women surveyed, 24.5 percent estimated that these rites cause long-term complications from urinary tract infections and 23.8 percent recognized that the rituals had caused chronic pelvic infection.

As high as the rate of these reported complications are, investigator El Dareer believes that the actual rates are probably even higher for several reasons. First, there are unenforced laws against female genital cutting. Although it is nonetheless widely practiced, people are reluctant to discuss illegal activities. Second, people may be ashamed to admit that they have had complications, fearing they are to blame. Third, some women believe that female circumcision or infibulation is necessary for their health and well-being and may not fully associate these problems with the surgery. They assume that their problems would have been worse without it. Of course, many other women, as these studies show, are well aware of the complications from these rituals.

Reasons for Female Genital Cutting

Investigators have identified five primary reasons for these rites: (1) religious requirement, (2) group identity, (3) cleanliness and health, (4) virginity, family honor, and morality, and (5) marriage goals, including greater sexual pleasure for men. These investigators, who are members of cultures practicing female genital mutilation, report many factual errors and inconsistent beliefs about the procedure and the goals they believe these rites serve. They therefore argue that the real reasons for continuing this practice in their respective countries rest on ignorance about reproduction and sexuality and, furthermore, that these rites fail as means to fulfill established community goals.

Meets a Religious Requirement According to these studies, the main reason given for performing female genital cutting and infibulation is that it is a religious requirement. Most of the people practicing this ritual are Muslims, but it is not a practice required by the Koran. El Dareer writes that "there is nothing in the Koran to suggest that the Prophet [Mohammed] commanded that women be circumcised." Female genital cutting and infibulation, moreover, is not practiced in the spiritual center of Islam, Saudi Arabia. Another reason for questioning this as a Muslim practice is that clitoridectomy and infibulation predate Islam, going back to the time of the pharaohs. . . .

Preserves Group Identity Investigators Koso-Thomas, El Dareer, and Abdalla agree that people in these countries support female circumcision as a good practice, but only because they do not understand that it is a leading cause of sickness, or even death, for girls, mothers, and infants, and a major cause of infertility, infection, and maternal-fetal complications. They conclude that these facts are not confronted because these societies do not speak openly of such matters. Abdalla writes, "There is no longer any reason, given the present state of progress in science, to tolerate confusion and ignorance about reproduction and women's sexuality."...

Helps to Maintain Cleanliness and Health The belief that the practice advances health and hygiene is incompatible with stable data from surveys done in these cultures, where female genital mutilation has been linked to mortality or morbidity such as shock, infertility, infections, incontinence, maternal-fetal complications, and protracted labor. The tiny hole generally left to allow for the passage of blood and urine is a constant source of infection. Koso-Thomas writes, "As for cleanliness, the presence of these scars prevents urine and menstrual flow from escaping by the normal channels. This may lead to acute retention of urine and menstrual flow, and to a condition known as *hematocolpos, which is highly detrimental to the health of the girl or woman concerned and causes odors more offensive than any that can occur through the natural secretions.*"...

Although promoting health is given as a reason for female genital mutilation, many parents seem aware of its risks and try to reduce the morbidity and mortality by seeking good medical facilities. Some doctors and nurses perform the procedures for high fees or because they are concerned about the unhygienic techniques that traditional practitioners may use. In many parts of the world, however, these practices are illegal, and medical societies prohibit doctors and nurses from engaging in them even if it might reduce morbidity and mortality.

Preserves Virginity and Family Honor Type 3 circumcision and infibulation is used to control women's sexual behavior by trying to keep women from having sexual intercourse before marriage or conceiving illegitimate children. In addition, many believe that types 2 and 3 circumcision are essential because uncircumcised women have excessive or even uncontrollable sexual drives. El Dareer, however, believes that this view is not consistently held in her culture, the Sudan, where women are respected and men would be shocked to apply this cultural view to members of their own families.

Beliefs that uncircumcised women have uncontrollable sexual drives, moreover, seem incompatible with the general view that sex cannot be pleasant for women, which investigators El Dareer, Koso-Thomas, and Abdalla found was held by both men and women in these cultures. Investigators also found that female circumcision and infibulation did not represent a foolproof way to promote chastity. These procedures can actually lead to promiscuity because they do not diminish desire or libido, even though they make orgasms impossible. Some women continually seek experiences with new sexual partners because they are left unsatisfied in their sexual encounters. Some even pretend to be virgins by getting stitched up tightly again.

Furthers Marriage Goals Those practicing female genital cutting not only believe that it promotes marriage goals, including greater sexual pleasure for men, but that it deprives women of nothing important, according to investigator Koso-Thomas. El Dareer and Abdalla also found widespread misconceptions that women cannot have orgasms and that sex cannot be directly pleasing to women coexisting with beliefs that these rites are needed to control women's libido and keep them from becoming "man-crazy."

To survive economically, women in these cultures must marry, and they will not be acceptable marriage partners unless they have undergone this ritual surgery. It is a curse, for example, to say that someone is the child of an uncircumcised woman. The widely held belief that infibulation enhances women's beauty and men's sexual pleasure makes it difficult for women who wish to marry to resist this practice. They view uncut female genitals as ugly.

For those outside these cultures, beliefs that these rites make women more beautiful are difficult to understand, especially when surveys show that many women in these cultures attribute keloid scars, urine retention, pelvic infections, puerperal sepsis, and obstetrical problems to infibulation. . . .

Promote Education

Female genital cutting and infibulation cause disability, death, and disease among mothers, infants, and children. It leads to difficulty in consummating marriage, infertility, prolonged and obstructed labor, and increased morbidity and mortality. It strains the overburdened health care systems in developing countries where it is practiced with impunity. Investigators who have documented these health hazards come from these cultures but draw upon interculturally shared methods of discovery, evaluation, and explanation in concluding that female genital mutilation fails as a means to fulfill many of the cultural goals for which it is intended, other than control of female sexuality. Although many values are culturally determined and we should not impose moral judgments across cultures hastily, we sometimes seem to know enough to condemn practices such as female genital mutilation, war, pollution, oppression, injustice, and aggression. Conventionalist ethical relativism challenges this view, but a substantial burden of proof falls on upholders of this moral theory to show why criticisms of other cultures *always* lack moral authority. Because of the hazards of even type 1 circumcision, especially on children, many groups, including WHO [the World Health Organization] and the AMA [American Medical Association], want to stop all forms of ritual genital surgery on women. Unenforced bans have proven ineffective, however, since this still popular practice has been illegal in most countries for many decades. Other proposals by activists in these regions focus on fines and enforcement of meaningful legislation, but education of the harms of genital cutting and infibulation may be the most important route to stop these practices. Thus an effective means to stopping these practices may be to promote education.

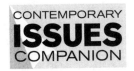

CHAPTER 2

Women and
Reproductive Health

The Risks of Fertility Treatments Are Unacceptable

Barbara Seaman

In 1978 Louise Brown, the first "test-tube baby," was born. As the result of the first successful in vitro fertilization (IVF), a procedure in which eggs taken from the mother are fertilized in a Petri dish and transferred into the womb, Louise's birth sparked thousands of physician-assisted conceptions. While many couples who had trouble conceiving welcomed this new development, many other people around the world raised ethical and safety concerns. A quarter of a century later, more women than ever are postponing families, thereby driving up the rate of assisted conception procedures undertaken each year. Barbara Seaman, well-known women's health journalist and activist, argues that these assisted reproductive procedures are taken too lightly and actually pose far more health risks than the public realizes. In the following selection she discusses the dangers of two of the most commonly used fertility drugs, Clomid and Lupron. Citing health experts and anecdotes from women who have used these drugs, she asserts that both drugs can lead to chronic and even fatal diseases, such as chronic physical distress and ovarian cancer. In addition to the potential health risks, Seaman points to the lack of live, healthy births as another disadvantage of seeking these fertility procedures and medications. She believes that the public is not made aware of these risks because drug companies and fertility clinics would lose far too much profit. Seaman is the author of several well-known books on women's health and medicine, including The Doctor's Case Against the Pill *and* The Greatest Experiment Ever Performed on Women: Exploding the Estrogen Myth.

Barbara Seaman, "Is This Any Way to Have a Baby?" *O Magazine*, February 2004. Copyright © 2004 by Barbara Seaman. Reproduced by permission of Georges Borchardt, Inc., on behalf of the author.

L ouise Brown [the world's first test-tube baby], now a postal worker in Bristol [England] celebrated her 25th birthday [in] July [2004]. And today fertility treatments are taken lightly, so much a part of our landscape that they're constant fodder for sitcoms like *Frasier* and *Friends*. But as the industry thrives at $2 billion a year, reproductive medicine is in many ways a Wild Wild West where doctors can practice like cowboys, using drugs that haven't been approved for fertility, and where no one is regulating the clinics, which often boast inflated success rates. "A fertility doctor can literally set up a lab in his garage and hire his son or daughter to run it, and it would be perfectly legal," says Brooks A. Keel, PhD, professor of biomedical sciences and associate vice president of research at Florida State University. "A woman gets more regulatory oversight when she gets a tattoo than when she gets IVF." Surprisingly, although the Clinical Laboratory Improvement Amendments of 1988 set strict quality control standards for medical laboratories, facilities that deal with women's eggs are exempt. Senator Ron Wyden of Oregon, who has steadily pushed for regulation of the fertility field, managed to get a bill passed in 1992 requiring that clinics at least report accurate success rates. But today some facilities notoriously cook their books to show the kind of success rates that will attract new patients. And Wyden himself acknowledges, "There is no question people still get around the law." By many accounts, government agencies like the Food and Drug Administration (FDA) and National Institutes of Health (NIH) are looking the other way. Fallout, perhaps, from politicized controversies over stem cell research and frozen embryos.

Painful Treatments

As almost any woman who has gone the fertility route knows, these treatments are often painful and always costly, and only one in four who attempt a test-tube pregnancy will take home a live baby, according to the best data available—odds that plunge to 5 percent at age 43 and only 2 percent after that. The grueling nature of even a single cycle is hard to grasp. "When I was on Gonal-F and Repronex, my abdomen got so swollen from the egg follicle production that I had difficulty breathing," says a woman named Mona P. who eventually did get pregnant with twins. "I gave myself subcutaneous injections in the stomach, and my husband gave the intramuscular injections in the hip. I hate needles. The night of egg retrieval, you take progesterone shots, which are extremely painful and create lumps under your skin. After retrieval my ovaries filled up with fluid, so I kept the uncomfortable bloated feeling for another three or four weeks. A horrible pain in my left shoulder lingered on and on. In all we paid $20,000 to the clinic, including about $4,000 for the drugs." Beyond discomfort, assisted reproductive techniques pose serious health threats like ectopic pregnancy (embryos may migrate or be inadvertently misplaced), and more than one out of three IVF deliveries are multiple births (which often result in childbirth complications and severe infant health problems). And it isn't just the physical trauma that lays women low, says Harvard professor Alice Domar, PhD, director of the Mind/Body Center for Women's Health at Boston IVF. It's also the rising disappointment with each treated cycle where hopes are raised, and then dashed. Without oversight of fertility clinics, many patients go through harrowing ordeals for nothing. I talked to some women who got the full monty [complete range] of ovulation hormones when they would later find out their husband's sperm was solely the problem, and others who were pumped with drugs before doctors realized their misshapen uteruses could never carry a fetus. In the absence of regulation, too, a rogue doctor is more likely to have free reign. . . .

But even with the best doctors and most sterling clinics, there are still glaring gaps in our knowledge about the danger fertility drugs may pose and whether the benefits outweigh the risks. A leading fertility scholar who prefers to remain anonymous minces no words: "This is a field that thrives in the absence of factual information. There is little work on animals to show safety, or randomized clinical trials to compare results. We make the same mistakes, but with increasing confidence." . . .

Clomid and Pergonal

The major drugs of concern in terms of ovarian cancer are those that induce ovulation, like Clomid, the typical first step for most infertile women, and Pergonal, which increases the number of eggs produced, and is often the second. Both were discovered in the 1950s, and for some infertile women, they're wonder drugs. Pergonal (human menopausal gonadotropin) is extracted from the urine of postmenopausal women and must be given by daily injection into the muscles of the buttocks or thighs. Clomid (clomiphene citrate, also sold as Serophene) can be taken orally. It is derived from DES (diethylstilbestrol), the infamous synthetic estrogen given to pregnant woman for 30 years before it was found, in the 1970s, to cause a rare form of cancer in their daughters, as well as birth defects like T-shaped uteruses and other anatomical distortions that make it difficult, if not impossible, to carry a baby.

Scientists theorize that the more often the ovaries are stressed by going through a monthly cycle ending in the rupture of an egg, the more prone they are to damage and to the development of abnormal cells that could become cancerous. Pregnancy and breastfeeding give your ovaries time off, and as a result, each child you have lowers your risk of ovarian cancer by 10 to 15 percent. Birth control pills, which suppress ovulation, are also known to decrease the cancer's frequency. Using this logic, hyperovulation caused by fertility drugs like Clomid and Pergonal would mean a higher risk.

In the early 1990s, two major studies linked such drugs to the occurrence of ovarian tumors, although in both cases the lead authors felt they had only shown enough evidence to warrant further investigation. Other studies failed to find a connection. In 2000, however, the well-respected Cochrane Collaboration, an independent organization that conducts reviews of medical studies, concluded that adverse effects of Clomid "include a possible ovarian cancer risk." Serono agrees that the relationship between its drug Serophene and ovarian cancer is "controversial" (the company also states that no causal link has been established for Pergonal). Dennis Marshall, PhD, executive director of medical affairs at Ferring, another fertility drug maker, notes that while there's no final answer on ovarian cancer, doctors are now using lower doses to stimulate patients' ovaries. . . .

Cancer and Other Health Risks

The journal *Fertility and Sterility* published an NIH study last year showing that women who took human menopausal gonadotropin (Pergonal-type drugs) for at least six cycles had a risk of breast cancer two to three times greater than women who had never used fertility medication. The findings are very tentative, but a few experts believe that breast—more than ovarian—cancer may emerge as the real concern. Cancer, however, is not the only cloud hanging over high-tech babymaking drugs. Any potential patient would think twice if she had sat next to Suzanne Parisian, MD, when this former FDA [Food and Drug Administration] official who wrote *FDA Inside and Out* studied the file of agency records on Lupron. A synthetic hormone that suppresses the pituitary gland, Lupron is often prescribed to both infertile women and egg donors to control the timing of ovulation. The drug, however, was never approved for this purpose. After writing a 100-page report, Parisian sent me a note: "Lupron is approved for only two short-term applications in women, (a) preoperative treatment of fibroids in patients with anemia and (b) management of endometriosis for a limit of six months. The FDA never approved Lupron for more than six months because there is significant risk of irreversible bone loss." Prescribing drugs for an unapproved, or "off-label," use is legal and quite common in medicine. But patients should be informed when it happens. And some women—especially "frequent fliers," who go through many cycles hoping for a baby—get more than the FDA's limit.

Parisian goes on to say that Lupron produces a postmenopausal state in women ("It literally drops the floor right out from beneath them without any time for the body to acclimate to the hormonal change"). Perhaps most alarmingly, she writes, far from being approved for fertility, Lupron "is 'pregnancy category X,' which means it is labeled not to be given to women intending to become pregnant or already pregnant. The entire IVF field uses Lupron for physician convenience. It lets them plan when to do [egg] harvests at a comfortable hour for them. They bully women into using it, telling them that there will be an increased risk of failure without Lupron. There is absolutely no real science to using Lupron for IVF."

. . .

A small percentage of women, it seems, never recover from what was supposed to be a temporary pituitary shutdown. At least one lawsuit filed on behalf of five Florida patients who took Lupron—for endometriosis and infertility—alleges that the drug causes chronic physical distress. TAP Pharmaceuticals denies liability for all the charges. More than a dozen women interviewed for this story, however, went on record to report a litany of medical complaints they believed to be the result of Lupron. Among the more common: autoimmune diseases, neurological problems, stomach disorders, and severe unexplained pain. Marriages fell apart. Careers languished. "We've gone to what seems like 5,000 doctors," laments the husband of one woman who at 25 was put on Lupron to help her get pregnant (she's since been hospitalized for chest pain and extreme hives, and suffers from a battery of other ailments). "They say, 'Think of something that might have caused all these things to suddenly come about.' And I tell them, 'Yeah! She took Lupron, and she's been sick ever since.' But they say Lupron doesn't have anything to do with it. I'm watching my wife fall apart in front of my eyes, and no one wants to do a thing about it." . . .

Profits Over Patient Safety

The push for effective fertility drugs has been fierce, fueled by the promise of pharmaceutical profits and by the collective ticking of America's biological clock, set ever later for having children. In 1970 Pergonal was still under study. That was the year that one volunteer, Margaret Kienast of New Jersey, gave birth to quintuplets. The publicity made infertile women frantic with hope. In Los Angeles Edward Tyler, MD (who happened to write for Groucho Marx on the side), had tried it on 300 patients but was still reluctant to recommend it for general use. The manufacturer, Cutter Laboratories, also believed the publicity was premature. One month after the Kienast births, the clinics testing Pergonal were booked solid and Tyler announced, "We don't have a vial in the house." Despite the hesitation of both the researchers and Cutter, the drug was approved that same year.

Today Pergonal has spawned a number of offshoots, including Humegon, Fertinex, Repronex, Gonal-F, and Follistim. In a recent interview, New Jersey fertility specialist Satty Gill Keswani, MD, (also a United Nations NGO delegate studying the environment's impact on fertility) described a close relative's near brush with death from a reaction to one of these ovulation drugs.

After trying to get pregnant for two years, Keswani's 34-year-old relative, "Danielle," was diagnosed with endometriosis. "Everything was okay except that one of her fallopian tubes was problematic," Keswani told me. She did not want Danielle to go ahead with IVF. "With one healthy tube, and being under 35, she still had a good chance without it," she said. "But many doctors press younger women to do IVF to increase their success numbers." Keswani does refer some of her own patients for IVF but notes that for those who fail after several tries, "it takes months to get the drugs out of their bodies." Keswani was attending a medical meeting in San Diego when Danielle, who had been on the ovulation drug for ten days, telephoned in tears. She had a pseudotumor in her brain. "This is a swelling that appears to be a tumor," Keswani says. "I ran for a plane and got home at 3 a.m. We did an MRI of her brain. The accumulated fluid of the pseudotumor had to be removed by spinal tap. I asked Danielle's doctors to stop the drug and showed them studies that it can cause blindness. The spinal fluid pressure was 480, when normally it would be 250. Her doctors, all men, wouldn't listen to me. They didn't want to 'interrupt the cycle' and let their treatment go to waste."

About 5 percent of patients taking this family of drugs develop hyperstimulation syndrome, which often involves the rapid enlargement of the ovaries and can be fatal. Fluid typically accumulates in the abdomen and sometimes the lungs, cutting off the breath; if the ovary ruptures, blood also pools and clots can occur. With Danielle, who fortunately survived, the excess fluid collected in the optic nerves. Two days after her spinal tap, doctors removed nine eggs, and when they had two or three embryos, they implanted them into her womb. It didn't work. "She was so down," Keswani tells me, "and it took three months for her eyes to clear up from the swelling of the nerves." But the story had a happy ending. Danielle and her husband went on vacation to Italy, says Keswani, "and they came back pregnant the good, old-fashioned way."

Lack of Informed Choice

If the risks of fertility drugs and treatments aren't clear, neither are the benefits. Add desperation for a child to the mix, and infertile women are in a difficult spot when it comes to making an informed choice about going high-tech.

Medical sociologist Joan Liebmann-Smith, PhD, a former board member of the patient advocacy group Resolve, calls the examining table where IVF is done "the gaming table" because when you go for treatment, you are literally taking a gamble. The real odds of taking a baby home, however, remain elusive. Even when clinics don't blatantly inflate their success rates, the industry is rife with a more subtle kind of manipulation that skews the final numbers. Ninety-three-year-old Howard Jones, MD, who cofounded the Jones Institute for Reproductive Medicine of Eastern Virginia Medical School, points out that busy clinics bent on posting stellar rates are apt to turn away the harder cases. Jane Miller, MD, a fertility doctor in New Jersey, agrees that smaller facilities and solo practitioners have a difficult time cracking the high numbers if they welcome the big-clinic rejects. The Society for Assisted Reproductive Technology tracks success rates of clinics for the Centers for Disease Control and Prevention (results can be seen at cdc.gov). But these figures, by and large, depend on the accuracy and honesty of the self-reporting clinics; most of which are the society's members.

Whether a woman needs help conceiving in the first place isn't always obvious. When she goes in for a workup, the specialist may have little incentive to send her back to the drawing board, or bed, as the case may be. "Bear in mind that if you wish to develop a reputation as a fertility doctor, you don't want patients getting pregnant on their own," as one insider puts it. Last May the Medical College of Georgia's distinguished authority Paul McDonough, MD, speaking to a group of New York and New Jersey fertility specialists, urged his colleagues to "go after the low-hanging fruit," meaning the obvious causes of infertility—sperm problems, fallopian tube injuries (from STDs and abortions), and genetic or prenatal conditions—before they pull out their prescription pads. Prospective patients might also consider patience. Some research shows that couples up to their mid-30s with no evident infertility factors have a better chance of success if they simply continue on their own.

The answers to all these questions will come one day. But for now, one can only proceed with extreme caution. For all the promise that reproductive medicine offers to those who dare to cross its threshold, with all the great joy it brings to a relatively small number of lucky seekers, it also breaks many hearts and bears risks that are yet unknown.

The Risks of Fertility Treatments Are Overstated

American Society of Reproductive Medicine

Following the appearance in O Magazine *of Barbara Seaman's article on the dangers of fertility treatments, a number of organizations responded to her assertions, claiming that her facts and citations are groundless and encourage women to fear reproductive treatments that are safe for the majority of patients. The American Society for Reproductive Medicine (ASRM), a national organization of reproductive specialists, issued such a statement. According to the ASRM, the evidence that Seaman uses in her article is dubious, and her major claims have been disproved by scientific studies. Specifically, the ASRM disputes her arguments that fertility drugs cause cancer and other serious medical conditions, that fertility doctors are not ethical and professional, and that the fertility industry is not regulated.*

ASRM is not in the habit of commenting on individual articles that appear in the lay press. While ASRM does not always agree with a journalist's perspective, we generally respect the integrity of their reporting and appreciate their genuine efforts to inform their readers. However, after publication of the article "Is This Any Way to Have a Baby?" in the February [2004] issue of *O Magazine*, we felt compelled to express our profound objections to the misstatements and implications in this article.

The article consists primarily of anecdotes from former infertility patients who either failed to become pregnant or had serious health issues during or following their infertility treatment. The manner in which these stories are presented

American Society of Reproductive Medicine, "Comments Regarding Article 'Is This Any Way to Have a Baby?' by Barbara Seaman, *O (Oprah) Magazine*, February 2004," *ASRM Bulletin*, vol. 6, January 29, 2004. Copyright © 2005 by ASRM. All rights reserved. Reproduced by permission.

implies that these tragic outcomes are common rather than the rare exception. The poorly researched reporting in this article can be appreciated from the citation of sources such as: "I talked to some women" and another as "A leading fertility scholar who prefers to remain anonymous said." No sincere effort is made to provide objectivity or to distinguish underlying medical problems that may be associated with but not caused by the infertility treatment. Therefore, ASRM believes that this particular situation warrants a response.

Patients often feel victimized by and angry about their infertility condition, particularly when treatments fail or are associated with physical and emotional discomfort. Rather than to provide useful, factual information, this article serves merely to mislead and frighten already vulnerable women and undermine their trust in their healthcare providers.

Rebuttals

ASRM would expect that a reputable magazine such as *O* would welcome and accept correction constructive criticism. ASRM would therefore like to provide the following rebuttal to this article:

1. *Fertility drugs cause cancer.* The photographs of two deceased celebrities (as the only two illustrations in the entire piece) would imply that ovarian cancer is a common, proven side effect of ovulation medications. Certainly, the exceptional accomplishments of these women underscore the tragedy of their early deaths. However, this conjecture is unsupported by any scientific data; in fact, the preponderance of the medical literature that has addressed this subject to date has found that ovulation medications do not increase the risk of either ovarian or breast cancer. Women who have never been pregnant are at the greatest risk of developing ovarian cancer. It is therefore logical that infertility is also a risk factor for ovarian cancer. While it is an attractive theory that excessive ovarian stimulation might increase the risk, numerous studies have

carefully scrutinized this possibility with none demonstrating an increased cancer incidence in patients exposed to infertility treatments. In fact, the Cochrane review cited by the author concludes that available data do not demonstrate a statistically significant increase in ovarian cancer associated with use of fertility medications.

The author implies that breast cancer may also be increased by fertility medications. Whereas conditions associated with an increased lifetime exposure to estrogen increase the risk of breast cancer, no studies have indicated that the very short-term estrogen elevation produced by fertility treatment increases breast cancer incidence.

2. *Fertility medications lead to ovarian hyperstimulation syndrome.* The case of a woman with a swollen abdomen and bloating after use of ovulation drugs is described in the article. Severe ovarian hyperstimulation syndrome is a serious and rare side effect of ovulation medications. Fortunately, this is largely avoided by the careful patient monitoring routine in IVF [in vitro fertilization] treatment. Less than 1% of all women undergoing assisted reproductive technologies develop severe hyperstimulation syndrome, although many will experience some bloating and ovarian discomfort. Patients undergoing IVF are routinely informed about this potential complication, and serious or long-term injury is exceedingly rare.

3. *IVF increases the risk of ectopic pregnancy.* The implication that IVF causes ectopic (tubal) pregnancy is extremely misleading. Infertility due to tubal disease is one of the most common indications for IVF, and patients with tubal factor infertility are at a high risk for ectopic pregnancy no matter how they conceive. In fact, the incidence of ectopic pregnancy after IVF in these women is *reduced* compared to spontaneous pregnancy.

4. *IVF is inappropriately recommended for patients with undiagnosed male infertility or abnormalities of the uterus.* The article implies that, among providers at ART (Assisted Repro-

ductive Technology) services, there is a general failure to appreciate sperm and uterine abnormalities that would preclude a successful pregnancy. It is the standard of care (applied by the overwhelming majority of IVF clinics) to evaluate both semen parameters and uterine anatomy prior to IVF treatment. In fact, IVF is the only successful treatment for severely compromised sperm number and/or function. Furthermore, IVF constitutes the only conclusive test of fertilization ability. While uterine abnormalities are frequently diagnosed in an infertility population, rarely are these abnormalities incompatible with pregnancy and delivery of a healthy child.

5. *Typical IVF practitioners are "rogue physicians".* For reasons that are not clear, the cases of two infertility physicians who were accused/convicted of criminal activity 10 and 15 years ago respectively were included in this article. As the lay reader should be able to appreciate, the implication that these reprehensible criminal activities are typical of fertility physicians in general is ludicrous.

6. *The use of Lupron for IVF leads to osteoporosis.* Lupron is a drug that suppresses the ability of the pituitary gland to stimulate the ovary. While the article alleges it is used in IVF for physician convenience, there is conclusive scientific evidence that use of use of a GnRH agonist such as Lupron increases the pregnancy rate compared to IVF cycles where these medications are not used. The most obvious advantage is that Lupron prevents ovulation from occurring before the eggs can be retrieved from the ovaries. The author focuses on the fact that this constitutes an "off label" use with regard to FDA approval. Such off label use of a drug for expanded indications is commonplace in medical practice, is recognized by the FDA, and routinely brings us new therapies for many diseases. The article implies that the use of Lupron for ovulation induction leads to irreversible bone loss (osteoporosis). This is a blatant example of the author's lack of understanding of the pharmacology and physiology of ovulation induction. When

used alone, Lupron results in low estrogen levels that over time (months to years) can lead to bone loss and osteoporosis. However, in the context of IVF, estrogen levels are suppressed very transiently (for a few days, similar to the duration that estrogen is low in normal menstrual cycles) followed by stimulation of the ovaries and rapid increase in the estrogen level that is more than sufficient to maintain bone density. Furthermore, there have been no reported cases of osteoporosis associated with Lupron in the context of IVF treatment.

7. *The fertility industry is not regulated.* Despite the author's statements to the contrary, the field of reproductive medicine is in fact heavily regulated. Physicians who specialize in infertility care, like all physicians, are licensed to practice by the states where they work. The Food and Drug Administration (FDA) approve all medications and devices used in the clinic. The FDA also requires all facilities that handle reproductive tissue to register with them, and has issued draft regulations for the handling of those tissues. Another federal agency, the Centers for Disease Control and Prevention (CDC) collect and report the outcomes from ART procedures from clinics throughout the country. This unique resource allows patients to examine the outcomes from each clinic one at a time. There is also extensive self-regulation by the profession. The Society for Assisted Reproductive Technology (SART) has extensive requirements for its members, including educational and certifications requirements for staff. The majority of infertility practitioners have undergone specialty training and board certification in Obstetrics and Gynecology, and many have completed additional subspecialty fellowship training and certification in Reproductive Endocrinology.

8. *Areas of Agreement.* There are three areas where we agree with the author: 1) patients have a right to accurate and current information about their fertility treatment; 2) it is the obligation of the health care provider to provide this informa-

tion and obtain patient consent for these elective treatments; and 3) we agree in the value of long-term, prospective studies to evaluate all aspects of the safety of ART for women and their children.

Pregnancy Concerns for Women over Age Thirty-Five

March of Dimes

As more and more women delay starting families until they are well into their thirties, forties, and even older, fertility treatments such as in vitro fertilization (IVF) and intrauterine insemination (IUI) have become more commonplace. For some experts, risks to an older mother and her fetus call into question not only the safety of such procedures but the ethics of using them as a method of achieving parenthood. In this selection the March of Dimes, a national organization devoted to the health and well-being of infants through research, support, and awareness, discusses the benefits and risks of pregnancy and birth in women over thirty-five. They begin by pointing out the decline in fertility after a woman reaches her mid-thirties. They also note that chronic health problems such as high blood pressure and diabetes are more commonly found in women over thirty-five, and these diseases should be monitored closely before, during, and after pregnancy to ensure the health of the mother and the baby. Birth defects, miscarriages, and pregnancy complications are also more likely to occur in women in their late thirties and beyond. Despite these increased risks, the March of Dimes asserts that it is possible for a woman over thirty-five to have a safe pregnancy and delivery if she is closely monitored and maintains a healthy lifestyle before and during the pregnancy.

Most women over age 35 have healthy pregnancies and healthy babies. Recent studies suggest, however, that older moms do face some special risks.

Since the late 1970s, birth rates for women in their late 30s and 40s have increased dramatically. According to the Na-

March of Dimes, "Pregnancy After 35," www.marchofdimes.com, November 2002. Copyright © 2005 by the March of Dimes Birth Defects Foundation. All rights reserved. Reproduced by permission.

tional Center for Health Statistics, between 1978 and 2000, the birth rates for women age 35 to 39 and 40 to 44 more than doubled.

Advances in medical care now help women in their late 30s and 40s have safer pregnancies than in the past. However, women should be aware of the risks associated with later childbearing so that they can make informed decisions about their pregnancies.

Age and Fertility

Women generally have some decrease in fertility starting in their early 30s. It is not unusual for a woman in her mid-30s or older to take longer to conceive than a younger woman.

Age-related declines in fertility may be due, in part, to less frequent ovulation or to problems such as endometriosis, in which tissue similar to that lining the uterus attaches to the ovaries or fallopian tubes and interferes with conception.

If conception has not taken place after six months of trying, a woman over age 35 should consult her health care provider. According to the American Society for Reproductive Medicine, about one-third of women between age 35 and 39 and two-thirds of women over 40 have fertility problems. Many cases of infertility can be treated successfully.

While women over age 35 may have more difficulty conceiving, they also have a greater chance of bearing twins. The likelihood of naturally conceived (without fertility treatment) twins peaks between ages 35 and 39.

Preexisting Health Problems

At any age, a woman should consult her health care provider before trying to conceive. A preconception visit helps ensure that she is in the best possible physical condition before conception.

This visit is a good time to discuss any concerns a woman and her partner may have about a pregnancy.

A preconception visit is especially important if a woman has a chronic health problem, such as diabetes or high blood pressure. These conditions, which are much more common in women in their late 30s and 40s than in younger women, can endanger the pregnant woman and her developing baby. Careful medical monitoring and appropriate choice of medications, started before conception and continued throughout pregnancy, can reduce the risks associated with these conditions and, in most cases, result in a healthy pregnancy.

Studies suggest that women over 35 are twice as likely as women in their 20s to develop high blood pressure and diabetes for the first time during pregnancy. A 1996 study at Mount Sinai School of Medicine in New York City found that women age 40 and older were almost three times as likely to develop diabetes, and almost twice as likely to develop high blood pressure as women in their 20s. Similarly, a 1999 study at the University of California at Davis found that first-time mothers over age 40 were 60 percent more likely to develop high blood pressure and four times more likely to develop diabetes during pregnancy than mothers in their 20s. This makes it especially important that older mothers get early and regular prenatal care. With early diagnosis and proper treatment, these disorders usually do not pose a major risk to mother or baby.

Birth Defects

The risk of bearing a child with certain chromosomal disorders increases as a woman ages. The most common of these disorders is Down syndrome, a combination of mental retardation and physical abnormalities caused by the presence of an extra chromosome 21 (humans have 23 pairs of chromosomes). At age 25, a woman has about a 1-in-1,250 chance of having a baby with Down syndrome; at age 30, a 1-in-1,000 chance; at age 35, a 1-in-400 chance; at age 40, a 1-in-100 chance; and at 45, a 1-in-30 chance.

The American College of Obstetricians and Gynecologists (ACOG) recommends that women with singleton pregnancies who will be 35 or older at the time of delivery should be offered prenatal testing (with amniocentesis or chorionic villus sampling) to diagnose or, more likely, rule out Down syndrome and other chromosomal abnormalities. About 95 percent of women who undergo prenatal testing receive the reassuring news that their baby does not have one of these disorders. If prenatal testing rules out chromosomal defects and the mother is healthy, the baby probably is at no greater risk of birth defects than if the mother were in her 20s.

Miscarriage Risks

Most miscarriages occur in the first trimester for women of all ages. The rate of miscarriage in older women is significantly greater than that in younger women. A 2000 Danish study found that about 9 percent of recognized pregnancies for women aged 20 to 24 ended in miscarriage. The risk rose to about 20 percent at age 35 to 39, and more than 50 percent by age 42. The increased incidence of chromosomal abnormalities contributes to the age-related risk of miscarriage.

Pregnancy Complications

While women in their late 30s and 40s are likely to have a healthy baby, they do face more complications along the way.

Besides the increased risk of diabetes and high blood pressure, women over 35 have an increased risk of placental problems. The most common placental problem is placenta previa, in which the placenta covers part or all of the opening of the cervix. The University of California at Davis study found that first-time mothers over age 40 were up to 8 times as likely as women in their 20s to have this complication. Placenta previa can cause severe bleeding during delivery, which can endanger mother and baby, but complications often can be prevented with a cesarean delivery.

Some studies suggest that women having their first baby at age 35 or older are at increased risk of having a baby who is low birthweight (less than 5½ pounds) or premature (born at less than 37 full weeks of pregnancy). A 2002 Canadian study found that women over age 35 were 20 to 40 percent more likely than younger women to have a low birthweight baby, and 20 percent more likely to have a premature delivery. These risks appear to rise modestly but progressively with a woman's age, even if she does not have age-related chronic health problems such as diabetes and high blood pressure.

The Danish study found that women over age 35 had an increased risk of ectopic pregnancy (in which the fertilized egg implants outside of the uterus, usually in the fallopian tube). The Danish and Canadian studies also found a slightly increased risk of stillbirth, though other studies did not.

The newborns of mothers in their 40s may suffer more complications (such as asphyxia and brain bleeds) than those of younger mothers, according to the University of California at Davis study. However, in spite of the increased risk of complications, there were no more deaths among babies of older mothers, and the vast majority of babies recovered and did fine.

Pregnant women who are 35 or older face some special risks, but many of these risks can be managed effectively with good prenatal care. It is important to keep in mind that the increased risk, even for the oldest women, is modest.

Problems with Labor and Delivery

First-time mothers over 35 are more likely than women in their 20s to have difficulties in labor. Studies suggest that fetal distress and a prolonged second stage of labor are more common in older mothers.

This may account, in part, for the increased rate of cesarean sections among women over 35. First-time mothers over age 40 have the highest risk of c-section, 43 percent, according to a 2001 study at Harvard Medical School in Boston. Similarly, other studies have reported that first-time mothers over age 35 have about a 40 percent chance of a c-section, compared to about a 14 percent risk for first-time mothers in their 20s.

Reducing Risks

Today, most women in their late 30s and 40s who are planning pregnancy can look forward to having a healthy pregnancy and a healthy baby. However, given the special concerns about pregnancy past age 35, it is especially important for older women to follow the basic rules for a healthy pregnancy:

- Plan for pregnancy by seeing a health care provider before you conceive. Medical conditions, medications and immunizations can be reviewed at this time.

- Take a multivitamin containing 400 micrograms of folic acid daily before you become pregnant and through the first month of pregnancy to help prevent neural tube defects. Get early and regular prenatal care.

- Eat a variety of nutritious foods, including foods containing folic acid, like fortified breakfast cereals, enriched grain products, leafy green vegetables, oranges and orange juice and peanuts. (Any woman with a history of nut allergies should avoid eating peanuts or peanut products at all times, not just while pregnant or breastfeeding.)

- Begin pregnancy at a healthy weight (not too heavy or too thin). Stop drinking alcohol before you try to conceive, and continue to avoid alcohol during pregnancy.

- Don't smoke during pregnancy and avoid secondhand smoke. It's best to quit before you become pregnant.

- Don't use any drug, even over-the-counter medications or herbal preparations, unless recommended by a health care provider who knows you are pregnant.

Controversies over Women's Access to Birth Control

Marcia Clemmitt

While arguments for and against the use of birth control pills have been around since before "the pill" first became available in the early 1960s, the controversy has recently gained new attention as reports about pharmacists refusing to fill birth control prescriptions make national headlines. Most of the controversy has focused on whether pharmacists have the right to morally object to filling these prescriptions. Another major issue of this debate focuses on emergency contraception, or the so-called "morning-after pill," which, if taken within seventy-two hours of sexual intercourse, may prevent conception. Marcia Clemmitt, a social-policy researcher and writer, attempts to sort out the current debate, which she refers to as "a new front in America's culture wars." She takes up several sides of the dispute, including religious and moral viewpoints, medical professionals' viewpoints, and women's viewpoints. In the end, she speculates, the disputes will be decided by the court system. Clemmitt is a former editor in chief of Health and Medicine *and is currently a staff writer for* CQ Researcher *in which this selection first appeared.*

Neil Noesen was filling in as a back-up pharmacist at the Menomonie, Wis., Kmart when college student Amanda Phiede came in to refill her prescription for birth-control pills.

Noesen is a devout Catholic who believes that birth-control pills can cause what he regards as early-stage abortions. Noesen—the lone pharmacist on duty that day—refused to fill Phiede's prescription.

"I explained to her that I couldn't give it to her with a good conscience," Noesen said. "I did not direct her to another pharmacy."

Phiede went to a nearby Wal-Mart, but when the pharmacist there asked Noesen to transfer her prescription, he refused. Two days later, the Kmart pharmacy manager—who had been out of town—finally filled Phiede's prescription. By then, she had missed a pill and had to take two pills to catch up, increasing her risk of unintended pregnancy. The incident occurred in 2002.

A state administrative board eventually charged Noesen with unprofessional conduct for refusing to transfer the prescription, which is considered the patient's property. In April 2005 the state pharmacy board ordered Noesen to attend ethics classes and pay about $20,000 to cover costs of the disciplinary proceedings. He was allowed to retain his pharmacy license as long as he informs all future employers in writing that he won't dispense birth-control pills and describes steps he will take to ensure that patients get their prescriptions some other way. . . .

Noesen has remained firm in refusing to have any part in dispensing birth control pills. Using the pills is "evil," under God's moral code, he told the disciplinary hearing last October. He would not transfer a contraceptive prescription because "it would be a sin to induce another to sin" and would make him "part of a bucket brigade, just another step in facilitating the end result."

Refusing to Dispense Contraception

Over the past several years, only a handful of pharmacists have refused to dispense contraception, and even fewer have tried to prevent a patient from obtaining pills elsewhere. Nevertheless, the incidents demonstrate that birth control has become a new front in America's culture wars. While recent battles have focused on abortion, debate over birth control has intensified—pitting the religious beliefs of a minority of Americans against the desire of the overwhelming majority to retain easy access to contraception.

According to a December 2004 report by the federal Centers for Disease Control and Prevention (CDC), contraceptive use in the United States "is virtually universal," with more than 98 percent of sexually active women of reproductive age having used "at least one contraceptive method" at some point.

Moreover, most doctors—including 87.5 percent of Catholic physicians—dispense birth control. Likewise, most healthcare providers and pharmacists generally support greater access, says Don Downing, a University of Washington professor of pharmacy. But many hospitals—especially those affiliated with the Roman Catholic Church, which make up a growing percentage of the hospitals in America—refuse to dispense contraceptives or emergency birth control, even to women who have been raped. The church opposes both birth control and abortion.

Emergency birth control consists of a large dose of regular birth-control pills that, when taken within five days after unprotected sex can prevent a pregnancy. Some religious conservatives and pro-life advocates object to it—as well as to regular birth-control pills and intrauterine devices—because they may interfere with a fertilized egg's implantation in the uterine wall. Opponents of such birth-control methods believe life begins when the egg is fertilized and that such pills and devices, in essence, cause the fertilized egg to be aborted.

But emergency contraception is not the only birth-control method stirring controversy. Some doctors, pharmacists and hospitals will not dispense or prescribe any birth control on the grounds that artificial contraception itself is wrong. Others object only to giving birth-control pills to single women who plan to use them for contraceptive purposes rather than for health reasons, such as regulating menstrual periods.

Health-care workers and hospitals that refuse on moral grounds to provide certain contraception services argue strongly that their constitutional right to religious freedom should protect them from employer sanctions, even if they refuse to refer patients elsewhere for birth control. "It [is] unethical to force practitioners to participate in specific actions involving what they believe would be a cooperation with abortions," Noesen told the Wisconsin legislature in 2003, when it was considering a conscience clause.

Opponents Face Off

Opponents of certain types of birth control and advocates for easy access to contraception are facing off in state legislatures across the country, as lawmakers debate a variety of bills governing contraceptives. Some states are considering mandating that hospitals and pharmacies dispense contraception—including emergency contraception—while other states are allowing health-care workers and hospitals to exercise their "conscience rights" not to dispense medications they see as facilitating abortions. Some states are trying to do both.

At least seven states—Alaska, California, Hawaii, New Hampshire, New Mexico, Washington and Maine—have allowed pharmacists to dispense emergency contraception (without having received a prescription from a doctor), as long as they collaborate with a local physician and follow a predetermined protocol. "Growing numbers of people are interested in dispensing [emergency contraception]," says Downing, who developed programs to enable pharmacists to dispense emergency birth control.

Meanwhile, the U.S. Food and Drug Administration (FDA) has been asked to allow over-the-counter sales of emergency contraceptives, called Plan B. In May 2004, the agency overruled its own scientific advisory panel, which had voted 23-4 in favor of Plan B. The agency said it agreed with the minority on the panel who argued there was not enough evidence that girls under 15 could safely take the product. The decision, which shocked birth-control advocates, was a significant victory for those opposed to emergency birth control on religious grounds.

Birth-control advocates point out that when pharmacists or hospitals refuse to dispense contraception—emergency or otherwise—it typically disadvantages those lacking easy transportation to another pharmacy or facility, most often the poor and women living in rural areas without alternative pharmacists or hospitals nearby.

Moreover, repeated federal cutbacks in family planning funds since 1998 also have disproportionately affected the poor, potentially leading to a jump in unintended pregnancies, says Carol Hogue, professor of maternal and child health at Emory University's Rollins School of Public Health. The cuts may already be reducing the use of birth control, she says, citing the CDC study, which showed that the number of adult women having unprotected sex during the previous three months rose from 5.2 percent in 1995 to 7.4 percent in 2002—the same level as in 1982. Low-income women rely heavily on subsidized birth control, and with government support waning, "it shouldn't be surprising that people aren't availing themselves of it as much," Hogue says.

Unintended Pregnancies

According to James Trussell, director of the Princeton University Office of Population Research, nearly half of unintended pregnancies (47 percent) occur among the small group of women who have unprotected sex. A 43 percent increase in that population recently reported by the CDC could create up to an 18 percent increase in unintended pregnancies, he says.

And more unintended pregnancies could lead to an increase in the number of abortions as well as "marital discord, domestic violence and children at high risk for developmental problems," Hogue points out.

But anti-contraception advocates argue that the same kinds of problems are triggered when birth control fails, as it often does. The result frequently is "abortion . . . single motherhood—often attended by poverty . . . or an unsuitable marriage that ends in divorce," says Janet Smith, chair of life ethics at Detroit's Sacred Heart Major Seminary and a well-known speaker on Catholic sexual ethics.

Religious Views, Not Science

Critics of the administration's birth-control policies say the FDA's refusal to allow Plan B—only the second time in 50 years the agency rejected an advisory panel's advice—was influenced more by the religious views of minority panel members than by science.

David Hager, an obstetrician-gynecologist and one of three panel members appointed by President [George W.] Bush, led the opposition to Plan B on the grounds that it may sometimes prevent implantation of a fertilized egg. He told FDA officials there was not enough evidence to show that nonprescription sales of Plan B would be safe for girls under 15. . . .

But the advisory panel's majority and many other analysts say Hager's assertion there is insufficient data on the safety of Plan B for young girls is not based on science at all. Trussell, a panelist who voted for over-the-counter sales, says the panel reviewed numerous studies showing that adolescents can understand Plan B's package instructions "as well as anybody else."

However, aside from questions about Plan B's appropriateness for young teens, the FDA also has dragged its heels in making Plan B available without a prescription for women over 16. A year ago, Barr Laboratories applied to sell Plan B over-the-counter to women 16 and older while requiring a prescription for girls under age 16. But the FDA let a January 2005 deadline to act on that application pass without taking action. Soon after that, Democratic Sens. Hillary Rodham Clinton (N.Y.) and Patty Murray (Wash.) announced they would hold up the confirmation of FDA Acting Commissioner Lester Crawford as commissioner until the FDA acts on Barr's new application.

In March Crawford told the Senate Health, Education, Labor and Pensions Committee that the decision has been slowed because "it's a very complex kind of application never received before by the agency."

Pharmacists Must Fill Prescriptions

Meanwhile, the American Medical Association [AMA] voted on June 20 to support legislative initiatives around the country requiring pharmacies to fill legally valid prescriptions.

If a pharmacist or pharmacy has objections, they should provide an "immediate referral to an appropriate alternative dispensing pharmacy without interference," said a resolution by the AMA's policymaking House of Delegates.

"Our position is on behalf of the patient," said Peter Carmel, an AMA board member and neurosurgeon from New Jersey. "The AMA strongly believes patients have to have access to their medications. It's the obligation on behalf of the pharmacist . . . to tell them where to go."

The AMA's policy would be similar to that of the nation's largest pharmacy chain, Walgreen Co. . . .

Should Religion Count?

The question is especially complicated in the case of emergency contraception, because it is only effective if taken within about five days of the unprotected intercourse.

Thus, refusing to fill a prescription "may place a disproportionately heavy burden on those with few options, such as a poor teenager living in a rural area that has a lone pharmacy," lawyer Julie Cantor and physician Ken Baum wrote last year in *The New England Journal of Medicine*. "A refusal to fill a prescription for a less advantaged patient may completely bar her access to medication."

It's also unclear where conscientious objection would end, once permitted. The consequences could amount to "invasive" behavior, according to Cantor and Baum. "If pharmacists can reject prescriptions that conflict with their morals, someone who believes that HIV-positive people must have engaged in immoral behavior could refuse to fill those prescriptions," they point out.

Achieving Balance

Many analysts agree that pharmacists' right to follow their consciences must be balanced against patients' right to have legal medications. But when it comes to achieving that balance, different people use different scales.

The issue is almost always framed as one of honoring—or not honoring—the pharmacist's conscience. But, says Rosemarie Tong, distinguished professor in health-care ethics at the University of North Carolina at Charlotte, there are always at least two consciences involved—the pharmacist's and the patient's. "Whose moral decision should be captive to the other person's in this situation?" she asks.

According to Tong, the person who risks less potential harm should yield right of conscience. In the case of emergency contraception, "the person who's going to bear the brunt of the pregnancy" risks harm that's "much greater" than the potential damage to a pharmacist who reluctantly violates his or her conscience.

Proponents of strong conscience clauses disagree. A woman seeking emergency contraception generally has plenty of other options, says physician David Stevens, executive director of the 17,000-member Christian Medical and Dental Associations. "Sign up for mail order, get a referral to another pharmacy," he suggests. But the pharmacist has only one conscience, and "conscience is the most sacred of all property."

Others argue that, given today's nationwide pharmacist shortage, druggists have more options. "What happens to the patient if a pharmacist has the right to refuse?" asks Todd Brown, an associate clinical specialist at the Northeastern University School of Pharmacy in Boston.

For pharmacists seeking so-called conscience clauses to protect them from employer retaliation if they refuse to dispense a drug, the issue hinges on whether they are going to be treated like professionals, says Noesen. Enacting a conscience clause "would simply be giving legal recognition to the professional autonomy that we already hold as pharmacists."

Limits of Professional Autonomy

But critics counter that professional autonomy is limited by the requirement that a pharmacist put the clients' needs first. "Professional autonomy has its limits," write Cantor and Baum. Pharmacy professionals "are expected to exercise special skill and care to place the interests of their clients above their own interest."

"I don't think pharmacists should have conscience clauses," Brown says. "They're not being asked to be the patient's religious leader."

Besides, he says, student pharmacists learn early on about the various kinds of medications provided by the health system. They should decide right away whether they object to dispensing them, says Brown, and those who have moral objections should work at pharmaceutical companies, health plans, nursing homes, hospitals and elsewhere, he says, rather than working in a pharmacy serving the general public.

But those calling for broad conscience clauses say it's very difficult to predict future medical treatments. As biomedical science advances, emergency contraception represents only the "tip of the iceberg" when it comes to technologies that may be morally objectionable, Stevens says. Other morally questionable therapies include stem cells and euthanasia drugs.

Supporting Conscience Clauses

The American Pharmacists Association (APhA) supports conscience clauses but thinks refusing pharmacists should refer customers to another pharmacist who will fill the prescription. When a pharmacist conscientiously objects, it is "appropriate to step away but not to step in the way," says Anne Burns, APhA's group director of pharmacy practice and research.

Individual employees' conscience objections should be discussed up front so a drug store—or an entire community—may put systems in place to protect pharmacists' conscience objections as well as patients' rights to get legal medications, Burns says. For example, "in rural areas, physicians could dispense" controversial drugs, she says.

But some health-care providers would consider that "moral complicity," Stevens says. . . .

States Conflicted over "Morning After" Pills

The introduction of emergency contraception pills into the U.S. market in 1998 injected new urgency into birth-control debates. Some providers have refused to dispense the pills, even to rape victims, claiming they cause early-stage abortions. The availability of a convenient pill that could protect rape victims from pregnancy and reverse birth-control mishaps like condom failure galvanized advocates to fight for wide availability.

State legislatures, where most of the current battles over emergency birth control are taking place, are pulled in two directions on the issue—as recent debates in Illinois and Colorado show.

Early this year, the Colorado legislature approved a bill allowing health-care professionals to refuse to offer emergency contraception due to religious or moral beliefs but requiring hospital emergency departments to offer rape victims information and referrals for obtaining emergency contraception.

Gov. Owens vetoed the measure in April, however, complaining that it did not offer protections to hospitals and other health-care institutions. "That is wrong," he said. "And it is unconstitutional."

As a testament to lawmakers' ambivalence, when sponsors led a failed attempt to override Owens' veto, several who had voted originally for the legislation later switched sides to vote against it.

Illinois, on the other hand, has the nation's most sweeping conscience law for health-care providers as well as the most liberal law in the nation regarding emergency contraception—a law requiring all pharmacies to dispense emergency contraception. Several Illinois pharmacists are suing Democratic Gov. Rod Blagojevich over the rule, arguing that it conflicts with the state's broad conscience exemption.

Public Opinion

If sheer numbers of supporters determined policy outcomes, laws broadening contraceptive access would be the easy winner. In a May 2005 poll, 73 percent of Americans said they believe pharmacists should be required to fill prescriptions for emergency contraception, even if they are personally opposed to it.

Nevertheless, arguments based on America's constitutional tradition of religious freedom, combined with conservative Christians' new political clout, have won a hearing for expanded conscience clauses—both in Congress and in statehouses around the country. . . .

Despite all the rhetoric over limiting access to birth control, states generally have considered more pro-birth control measures recently than efforts to limit access to contraception. . . .

Courts to Decide?

The strong public desire for contraceptive access, coupled with the growing strength of Christian conservatives in American life, promises to fuel birth-control debates into the foreseeable future, says Allan Rosenfield, an obstetrician-gynecologist and dean of Columbia University's Mailman School of Public Health. High-level political opposition to birth control "is not something that's going to go away without changing not only the administration but Congress as well, and I don't see that happening," he says.

Ultimately, the disputes will be decided by the courts, says ethicist Tong at the University of North Carolina. For instance, pharmacists in Illinois are suing the governor over the rule requiring pharmacies to dispense emergency contraception, arguing that it conflicts with Illinois' broad conscience clause.

Judicial settlements deal in the "limited language of rights" and don't necessarily deal with the full scope of these delicate issues, since they "opt out of the emotional tangles" involved, Tong says. Nevertheless, "only the courts can untangle whose conscience trumps whose," a provider's or a patient's.

Stress Negatively
Impacts Fertility

Lori Oliwenstein

Treatment for infertility can be extremely difficult both physi-
cally and psychologically. In this selection, Lori Oliwenstein dis-
cusses recent insights into these treatments that reveal that stress
can play a large role in their success or failure. Women (and to
some extent men) under stress have lower chances of conceiving
than their calmer counterparts. Unfortunately, there is no evi-
dence proving that treatment of the underlying stress increases
rates of conception. It is recommended that women with a his-
tory of mood disorders such as anxiety and depression seek treat-
ment for these disorders before they attempt infertility treatment.
Oliwenstein is a science writer and the author of Taming Bipolar Disorder.

Patricia and Derek couldn't have chosen a worse time to
begin trying to conceive. Derek's sister had just died, completely unexpectedly. Still, it was that event that pushed them
to make up their minds in the first place.

Though stressful, "it was a crystallizing moment for both
of us," Patricia recalls.

But after nine months of trying, the couple sought out a
fertility specialist and began a regimen of treatment that mil-
lions of women are currently undergoing, many in its most
high-tech form, in vitro fertilization (IVF).

"Each month was another cycle of stress and depression,"
Patricia recalls. "Do the meds, do the drugs, do the blood
tests, have the ultrasound, have sex, wait for test results, do
the meds, do the drugs. . . . Then you get your period, and it
is like a death. But you only have a few hours to grieve before
you have to start the pills and the needles and the tests again."

Lori Oliwenstein, "On Fertile Ground," *Psychology Today*, vol. 38, November/December
2005. Copyright © 2005 by Sussex Publishers, Inc. Reproduced by permission.

After three months, Patricia was both literally and figuratively sick and tired of the process—and more stressed than ever. When their physician suggested the couple take a break before considering the next step, Derek and Patricia knew it was the right thing to do.

"After two months of being off any treatments, I was still feeling sick: weak, fatigued, nauseated," Patricia says. "I was pretty frustrated, so I called my doctor to ask when we might resume treatment. She asked when my last period was, and I told her I still hadn't gotten a period since our last failed treatment in early June."

Andy—Patricia and Derek's son, conceived during their very first "off-treatment" cycle—was born in April of 1997.

Patricia and Derek's story is the kind that will likely make anyone wince who has wrestled with fertility issues. If you've tried to become pregnant and had even the slightest hint of trouble, you've probably been told one or two—or a dozen—similar tales, most of which end with the clichéd assertion that if you want to get pregnant all you have to do is stop trying so hard and relax. It's enough to make you want to strangle someone.

According to the American Society for Reproductive Medicine, well over 6 million Americans—about 10 percent of those of reproductive age—struggle with infertility, which is defined as not being able to achieve a pregnancy after trying for 12 months (six, if you're a woman 35 or over). Those aren't the most encouraging numbers, but what is perhaps most disturbing about them is that you rarely know ahead of time whether they do or don't, will or won't, apply to you.

A Viscious Cycle

For many couples who have decided to try to begin or expand their family, that means each month's hastily unwrapped negative pregnancy test brings with it a little more stress, a little more disappointment, a little more guilt—and maybe a lot more depression. But a growing body of evidence suggests that those feelings may tip the mind-body balance so that the next test is negative again. The question is, just how vicious is this particular cycle?

As Patricia discovered, a low mood is linked to low fertility. "Research shows that a woman who has a history of depression is twice as likely to subsequently experience infertility as a woman with no history of depression," says Alice Domar, director of the Mind/Body Center for Women's Health at Boston's Beth Israel Deaconess Medical Center.

It's no better at the other end of the street. Domar cites surveys showing that women who are infertile are as stressed-out as those who suffer from cancer, AIDS or heart disease.

Widely considered the preeminent expert on the relationship between mood and fertility, Domar has herself conducted studies showing that the more stressed a woman is, the less likely she is to achieve pregnancy with the higher-tech infertility treatments, like IVF. Even more compelling, she's demonstrated that when women are taught a meditative practice known as the "relaxation response" along with visualization, yoga and participate in support groups, the likelihood of pregnancy rises sharply.

Others have highlighted a link between the stress of infertility treatment and the outcome of that treatment. Depression, for example, is associated with high rates of dropout from infertility treatment.

In fact, emotional stress is the second-most frequently cited reason for dropping out of infertility treatment, trailing only financial constraints. It's not that the treatments are difficult, but that the people undergoing them simply can't take the conception-related pressure for long. In one Swedish study, a group of couples having trouble conceiving was offered three free cycles of IVF. Fifty-four percent dropped out of the program before completing all three cycles. The reason most commonly given was psychological stress. In an Australian study, couples offered six free IVF cycles completed only 3.1, on average; again, stress and mood effects were the top reasons cited for dropping out.

When treatment and its attendant stresses stop, pregnancy occurs often enough to be a documented phenomenon. A 2004 study from the Netherlands found that 26 percent of women who chose to drop out of fertility treatment after their first cycle went on to become pregnant without further treatment. Thirteen percent of women who dropped out after the second treatment cycle also became pregnant afterward.

Exactly how perceived stress results in reduced fertility is still sketchy, but the links in the chain of causation are becoming clearer. Negative emotions can kick stress hormones like cortisol into overdrive. Those stress hormones, in turn, alter physiology in ways that can be at odds with conception—by lengthening the menstrual cycle, for instance.

Men, Stress, and Infertility

While women shoulder most of the burden of fertility-related stress, it is not theirs exclusively. Men experiencing psychological distress tend to produce less ejaculate with fewer sperm and lower motility. In a recent study of more than 800 couples followed over 12 months, researchers from the United Kingdom and Denmark showed that stress in men—in particular, personal and marital stresses—led to a lower likelihood of achieving pregnancy via infertility treatment.

Still, the impact of male stress on fertility is much weaker than is the impact of female stress. The external pressures placed on men to reproduce are significantly less than those placed on women, and their response to those stresses is correspondingly less intense.

An evolutionary perspective provides added logic. Stress creates an inhospitable environment for sustaining a pregnancy. Stress hormones signal the presence of some kind of external crisis—and a crisis does not supply the most advantageous conditions for sustaining a pregnancy for nine months. A body that is receiving a constant barrage of distress signals does not put its main focus on pouring time and energy into conception.

Men, as the Danish researchers recently pointed out, "contribute to conception but not to actual pregnancy, limiting the time interval in which their emotions can influence the biological event relative to women." While a woman's mood can influence everything from fertilization to implantation to fetal growth, a man's mood plays a role only in the production and delivery of sperm.

Just how important mood is in men and women is itself unclear: a fact that will frustrate some and buoy others.

Conflicting Evidence

As recently as August [2005], a study in the journal *Human Reproduction* disputed Domar's findings that stress diminishes the effectiveness of IVF. It followed 166 women from before they began IVF to right before egg retrieval. The researchers searched for some factor that could discriminate between those who later conceived during that particular cycle and those who didn't. They found none.

Teasing out a link between mood and fertility is even more difficult when researchers look not at people undergoing high-tech infertility treatments but at the mass of humanity simply setting out to try to conceive a child the old-fashioned way.

"Do I think that mood plays a critical role in conceiving?" asks Kris Bevilacqua, a psychologist at New York's Montefiore Institute for Reproductive Medicine and Health. "Yes and no. No, because women who are raped conceive. And yes, because when couples are in a good mood, feeling positive and optimistic, it helps them go further, try a little harder."

Just Relax

Where does that leave you? Domar's studies suggest that mood influences the success of infertility treatment. But no data show that the treatment of psychological distress leads to any rise in pregnancy rates among the general population.

And as for all those people who tell you "just relax, you'll get pregnant in no time," they don't really have a clue what they're talking about, notes William Petok, chairman of the mental health group of the American Society of Reproductive Medicine. "Besides, I've never met anybody to whom you could say, 'Just relax,' and they'd do it. So it's bad advice."

And to whom does it even apply? "Most couples do not begin their reproductive efforts with feelings of depression and anxiety," observes Madeline Licker Feingold, director of psychological services at Alta Bates In Vitro Fertilization Program in Berkeley, California. "In fact, most people take fertility for granted—usually having spent many years guarding against an unplanned pregnancy—and begin the process of family building with hope, joy and excitement. Then they are shocked to learn of their infertility and often torment themselves for wasting time with birth control and waiting too long to try to conceive."

If you have a history of depression or anxiety, it would be wise to talk to a doctor, Domar advises. "I recommend that anyone who wants to get pregnant get their distress level under control before even trying to conceive."

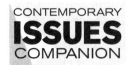

CONTEMPORARY
ISSUES
COMPANION

CHAPTER 3

Women and
Mental Health

Women Are at a Greater Risk of Depression than Men

National Institute of Mental Health

According to the World Health Organization (WHO), depression is the leading cause of disability in the United States and worldwide. Although depression varies from person to person, studies show that women are twice as likely to experience depression than men, regardless of racial, ethnic, or economic status. A study by the National Institute of Mental Health (NIMH) points to biology, life cycle, and psycho-social dimensions to account for this dramatic difference between women and men. As excerpted in the following selection, this study highlights seven specific causes for depression in women: issues occurring in adolescence, stressful situations at home and at work, reproductive events (menstruation, pregnancy, infertility, and menopause), cultural issues, victimization and abuse, poverty, and losing a spouse later in life. The NIMH is one of twenty-seven subdivisions of the National Institutes of Health and conducts research on psychological and behavioral disorders.

Life is full of emotional ups and downs. But when the "down" times are long lasting or interfere with your ability to function, you may be suffering from a common, serious illness—depression. Clinical depression affects mood, mind, body, and behavior. Research has shown that in the United States about 19 million people—one in ten adults—experience depression each year, and nearly two-thirds do not get the help they need. Treatment can alleviate the symptoms in over 80 percent of the cases. Yet, because it often goes unrecognized, depression continues to cause unnecessary suffering.

Depression is a pervasive and impairing illness that affects both women and men, but women experience depression at

National Institute of Mental Health, "Depression: What Every Woman Should Know," www.nimh.nih.gov, 2000.

roughly twice the rate of men. Researchers continue to explore how special issues unique to women—biological, life cycle, and psychosocial—may be associated with women's higher rate of depression.

No two people become depressed in exactly the same way. Many people have only some of the symptoms, varying in severity and duration. For some, symptoms occur in time-limited episodes; for others, symptoms can be present for long periods if no treatment is sought. Having some depressive symptoms does not mean a person is clinically depressed. For example, it is not unusual for those who have lost a loved one to feel sad, helpless, and disinterested in regular activities. Only when these symptoms persist for an unusually long time is there reason to suspect that grief has become depressive illness. Similarly, living with the stress of potential layoffs, heavy workloads, or financial or family problems may cause irritability and "the blues." Up to a point, such feelings are simply a part of human experience. But when these feelings increase in duration and intensity and an individual is unable to function as usual, what seemed a temporary mood may have become a clinical illness.

The Types of Depressive Illness

1. In major depression, sometimes referred to as unipolar or clinical depression, people have some or all of the symptoms listed below for at least 2 weeks but frequently for several months or longer. Episodes of the illness can occur once, twice, or several times in a lifetime.

2. In dysthymia, the same symptoms are present though milder and last at least 2 years. People with dysthymia are frequently lacking in zest and enthusiasm for life, living a joyless and fatigued existence that seems almost a natural outgrowth of their personalities. They also can experience major depressive episodes.

3. Manic-depression, or bipolar disorder, is not nearly as common as other forms of depressive illness and involves disruptive cycles of depressive symptoms that alternate with mania. During manic episodes, people may become overly active, talkative, euphoric, irritable, spend money irresponsibly, and get involved in sexual misadventures. In some people, a milder form of mania, called hypomania, alternates with depressive episodes. Unlike other mood disorders, women and men are equally vulnerable to bipolar disorder; however, women with bipolar disorder tend to have more episodes of depression and fewer episodes of mania or hypomania. . . .

Women Are at Greater Risk for Depression than Men

Major depression and dysthymia affect twice as many women as men. This two-to-one ratio exists regardless of racial and ethnic background or economic status. The same ratio has been reported in 10 other countries all over the world. Men and women have about the same rate of bipolar disorder (manic-depression), though its course in women typically has more depressive and fewer manic episodes. Also, a greater number of women have the rapid cycling form of bipolar disorder, which may be more resistant to standard treatments.

A variety of factors unique to women's lives are suspected to play a role in developing depression. Research is focused on understanding these, including: reproductive, hormonal, genetic or other biological factors; abuse and oppression; interpersonal factors; and certain psychological and personality characteristics. And yet, the specific causes of depression in women remain unclear; many women exposed to these factors do not develop depression. What is clear is that regardless of the contributing factors, depression is a highly treatable illness.

The Many Dimensions of Depression in Women

Investigators are focusing on the following areas in their study of depression in women:

The Issues of Adolescence Before adolescence, there is little difference in the rate of depression in boys and girls. But between the ages of 11 and 13 there is a precipitous rise in depression rates for girls. By the age of 15, females are twice as likely to have experienced a major depressive episode as males. This comes at a time in adolescence when roles and expectations change dramatically. The stresses of adolescence include forming an identity, emerging sexuality, separating from parents, and making decisions for the first time, along with other physical, intellectual, and hormonal changes. These stresses are generally different for boys and girls, and may be associated more often with depression in females. Studies show that female high school students have significantly higher rates of depression, anxiety disorders, eating disorders, and adjustment disorders than male students, who have higher rates of disruptive behavior disorders.

Adulthood: Relationships and Work Roles Stress in general can contribute to depression in persons biologically vulnerable to the illness. Some have theorized that higher incidence of depression in women is not due to greater vulnerability, but to the particular stresses that many women face. These stresses include major responsibilities at home and work, single parenthood, and caring for children and aging parents. How these factors may uniquely affect women is not yet fully understood.

For both women and men, rates of major depression are highest among the separated and divorced, and lowest among the married, while remaining always higher for women than for men. The quality of a marriage, however, may contribute significantly to depression. Lack of an intimate, confiding relationship, as well as overt marital disputes, have been shown to be related to depression in women. In fact, rates of depression were shown to be highest among unhappily married women.

Reproductive Events Women's reproductive events include the menstrual cycle, pregnancy, the postpregnancy period, infertility, menopause, and sometimes, the decision not to have children. These events bring fluctuations in mood that for some women include depression. Researchers have confirmed that hormones have an effect on the brain chemistry that controls emotions and mood; a specific biological mechanism explaining hormonal involvement is not known, however.

Many women experience certain behavioral and physical changes associated with phases of their menstrual cycles. In some women, these changes are severe, occur regularly, and include depressed feelings, irritability, and other emotional and physical changes. Called premenstrual syndrome (PMS) or premenstrual dysphoric disorder (PMDD), the changes typically begin after ovulation and become gradually worse until menstruation starts. Scientists are exploring how the cyclical rise and fall of estrogen and other hormones may affect the brain chemistry that is associated with depressive illness.

Postpartum mood changes can range from transient "blues" immediately following childbirth to an episode of major depression to severe, incapacitating, psychotic depression. Studies suggest that women who experience major depression after childbirth very often have had prior depressive episodes even though they may not have been diagnosed and treated.

Pregnancy (if it is desired) seldom contributes to depression, and having an abortion does not appear to lead to a higher incidence of depression. Women with infertility problems may be subject to extreme anxiety or sadness, though it is unclear if this contributes to a higher rate of depressive illness. In addition, motherhood may be a time of heightened risk for depression because of the stress and demands it imposes.

Menopause, in general, is not asssociated with an increased risk of depression. In fact, while once considered a unique disorder, research has shown that depressive illness at menopause is no different than at other ages. The women more vulnerable to change-of-life depression are those with a history of past depressive episodes.

Specific Cultural Considerations As for depression in general, the prevalence rate of depression in African American and Hispanic women remains about twice that of men. There is some indication, however, that major depression and dysthymia may be diagnosed less frequently in African American and slightly more frequently in Hispanic than in Caucasian women. Prevalence information for other racial and ethnic groups is not definitive.

Possible differences in symptom presentation may affect the way depression is recognized and diagnosed among minorities. For example, African Americans are more likely to report somatic symptoms, such as appetite change and body aches and pains. In addition, people from various cultural backgrounds may view depressive symptoms in different ways. Such factors should be considered when working with women from special populations.

Victimization Studies show that women molested as children are more likely to have clinical depression at some time in their lives than those with no such history. In addition, several studies show a higher incidence of depression among women who have been raped as adolescents or adults. Since far more women than men were sexually abused as children, these findings are relevant. Women who experience other commonly occurring forms of abuse, such as physical abuse and sexual harassment on the job, also may experience higher rates of depression. Abuse may lead to depression by fostering low self-esteem, a sense of helplessness, self-blame, and social isolation. There may be biological and environmental risk factors for depression resulting from growing up in a dysfunctional family. At present, more research is needed to understand whether victimization is connected specifically to depression.

Poverty Women and children represent 75 percent of the U.S. population considered poor. Low economic status brings with it many stresses, including isolation, uncertainty, frequent negative events, and poor access to helpful resources. Sadness and low morale are more common among persons with low incomes and those lacking social supports. But research has not yet established whether depressive illnesses are more prevalent among those facing environmental stressors such as these.

Depression in Later Adulthood At one time, it was commonly thought that women were particularly vulnerable to depression when their children left home and they were confronted with "empty nest syndrome" and experienced a profound loss of purpose and identity. However, studies show no increase in depressive illness among women at this stage of life.

As with younger age groups, more elderly women than men suffer from depressive illness. Similarly, for all age groups, being unmarried (which includes widowhood) is also a risk factor for depression. Most important, depression should not be dismissed as a normal consequence of the physical, social, and economic problems of later life. In fact, studies show that most older people feel satisfied with their lives.

About 800,000 persons are widowed each year. Most of them are older, female, and experience varying degrees of depressive symptomatology. Most do not need formal treatment, but those who are moderately or severely sad appear to benefit from self-help groups or various psychosocial treatments. However, a third of widows/widowers do meet criteria for major depressive episode in the first month after the death, and half of these remain clinically depressed 1 year later. These depressions respond to standard antidepressant treatments, although research on when to start treatment or how medications should be combined with psychosocial treatments is still in its early stages.

Depression Is a Treatable Illness

Even severe depression can be highly responsive to treatment. Indeed, believing one's condition is "incurable" is often part of the hopelessness that accompanies serious depression. Such individuals should be provided with the information about the effectiveness of modern treatments for depression in a way that acknowledges their likely skepticism about whether treatment will work for them. As with many illnesses, the earlier treatment begins, the more effective and the greater the likelihood of preventing serious recurrences. Of course, treatment will not eliminate life's inevitable stresses and ups and downs. But it can greatly enhance the ability to manage such challenges and lead to greater enjoyment of life.

Women Are More Susceptible to Developing Anxiety Disorders than Men

Susan Mahler

The roots of modern-day anxiety disorders such as generalized anxiety disorder (GAD), panic disorder, agoraphobia, and social phobia reach all the way back to the ancient Greek physician, Hippocrates, who attributed women's anxiety symptoms, such as nervousness, sweating, and heart palpitations, to hysteria, a condition in which the womb wanders in the body. Although this theory was finally debunked in the latter half of the twentieth century, Hippocrates' "wandering uterus" concept greatly impacted the research on and treatment of women's mental health for centuries. In the following selection, Susan Mahler begins with a discussion of this well-known history, connecting it to Sigmund Freud's psychoanalytic work with the hysteria phenomenon that was sweeping Victorian England and America during his lifetime. Mahler attempts to sort out the complexities of the causes of anxiety disorders and why women suffer from them two to three times more than men by separating the causes into two camps: nature versus nurture. Some researchers argue that changes in women's biological chemistry during menstruation, pregnancy, and menopause make them more susceptible to developing anxiety disorders. Researchers in the nurture camp, however, look to women's life experiences, such as their increased risk of sexual assault and their typical role as the family worrier, as the main reasons why women are more likely to suffer from anxiety disorders than men. Without treatment, notes Mahler,

Susan Mahler, "Anxiety Disorders," *The Complete Guide to Mental Health for Women*, edited by Lauren Slater, Jessica Henderson Daniel, and Amy Elizabeth Banks. Boston: Beacon Press, 2003. Copyright © 2003 by Beacon Press. All rights reserved. Reproduced by permission.

anxiety disorders are likely to persist and often coexist with other psychological disorders such as depression and addiction. Mahler is a writer and a psychiatrist working in the Boston area.

A woman sits at an oak desk, her loose-leafed papers spread before her in disarray. She wears a long nightdress and an anxious, distressed expression. She fidgets, sighs, bites her cuticle, gnaws her pencil. She is trying, failing, to fight off the attack of "nervous depression—a slight hysterical tendency" to which she is increasingly prone.

The woman in question is the nameless narrator in Charlotte Perkins Gilman's classic Victorian tale of female subordination, *The Yellow Wallpaper*. She might as well, though, be any one of us—the woman who appears in the glossy drug ad pages of the *American Journal of Psychiatry*, or the one in the television commercial, sitting with furrowed brow while a disembodied voice expounds on the curative properties of a certain medication.

A Brief History of Anxiety

For over a century, anxiety in various guises has been associated with women; not only is the psychological canon replete with anxious women, there is also a lengthy history of locating the cause in women's biology. *Hysteria* means, literally, "wandering uterus," and to this organ's intransigence the ancient Greeks ascribed a host of physical and mental symptoms. According to Hippocrates: "And if you then palpate the uterus, it is not in its proper place; her heart palpitates, she gnashes her teeth, there is copious sweat, and . . . they do all sorts of unheard-of things."

This anatomical view of hysteria persisted, with some variations, for over two millennia. With [Sigmund] Freud [the father of psychoanalysis], however, hysteria migrated from the physiological to the psychic realm. In *Dora: Analysis of a Case of Hysteria*, he posited that hysterical symptoms were caused by unconscious conflicts, that the symptoms themselves expressed those conflicts symbolically, and that treatment would entail making the unconscious conscious through analysis.

For Freud, the unconscious conflict in question was invariably a sexual one. Feminist revisionists, alternatively, have suggested that the manifestations of hysteria—the shortness of breath, palpitations, throat tightness, and weakness—were actually a vivid and accurate rendering of women's voicelessness and powerlessness.

Far apart though they may seem Freud and his critics agree on one thing: that anxious symptoms originate in the unconscious but are experienced all too consciously by both mind and body. This view of anxiety provides a framework for understanding a wide range of symptoms, from the heart-thumping intensity of a panic attack, to compulsive hand washing, to the fearful isolation of the agoraphobic. A century after Freud, neurobiologists are finding evidence that supports the role of the unconscious in producing anxiety. For instance, stimulation of the amygdala, a brain region associated with emotion and memory, produces a physiological response akin to panic without being precipitated by anything conscious. . . .

Causes of Anxiety

Interestingly, women remain two to three times more likely than men to develop anxiety disorders. What, if we dispense with the theory of uterine intransigence, can account for this difference? The theories set forth to explain the gender imbalance reflect the age-old debate between nature and nurture, between innate and acquired susceptibility to illness. According to the biological determinists, fluctuations in the level of estrogen at various times during a woman's life (menses, pregnancy, menopause), via effects on serotonin and other neurotransmitters, confer a predisposition to both mood and anxiety disorders. Evidence for this theory derives from epidemiological findings that symptoms of anxiety worsen premenstrually as well as postpartum (both periods associated with a rapid decline in estrogen levels). However, estrogen treatment of mood and anxiety disorders has not been conclusively shown to ameliorate symptoms, suggesting a more complex interaction between hormonal shifts and psychological illness.

Those in the biological camp also propose an evolutionary explanation for women's higher level of anxiety. Historically, women who were more vigilant, more closely attuned to their environments were more likely to protect themselves and their children. In this model, fear of certain environments (as in agoraphobia and Social Phobia) might have conferred survival value.

Nonsense, say those in the nurture camp. One need not look beyond women's life experience to explain their increased risk. They point to the increased risk of sexual abuse among women. In fact, women with a history of childhood physical or sexual abuse have a higher risk of both depression and anxiety and have a heightened adrenaline response—in other words, they are more physiologically "primed"—to mild stress.

These critics also note that anxiety is a more acceptable condition in women than it is in men. Women are likely to absorb the anxiety and fearfulness of their partners, becoming the family bearer of worry and tension. Finally, say the environmentalists, women's entry into the workplace spawned new anxieties about how to negotiate the balance between the personal and the professional. Two decades of feminist revisions to psychological theories have taught us that women develop in relation to others, and that for them, the work-world issues of success and competitiveness, self-esteem and competency can be fraught with difficulty. Surely, this transition alone could account for increased levels of psychological distress.

It is likely the case that all of these elements play a role in heightening women's risk of depression and anxiety, just as likely that we will never ferret out the precise contribution of each. Perhaps the best we can hope for is an awareness that anxiety disorders are complex, multifactorial conditions requiring an integrated approach to treatment.

Generalized Anxiety Disorder

Mrs. P., a forty-five-year-old court stenographer, presents to her primary care doctor for complaints of chronic muscle tension, difficulty sleeping, fatigue, and irritability. She has had difficulty concentrating at work and is short-tempered with her family. Her husband adds that she has "always been a worrier" and that she often seems overly distressed about things of minor importance.

The preceding case could describe a woman with depression, or one with any number of medical conditions. Most likely, however, is a diagnosis of Generalized Anxiety Disorder (GAD), a condition characterized by excessive anxiety and worry about a number of life events or circumstances. The subjective feeling of anxiety is accompanied by signs of physical distress; for this reason, many people first go to their family physicians for treatment. . . .

What sets GAD apart from run-of-the-mill worrying is that the degree of concern is excessive—out of proportion to the context—so that it causes the person distress and interferes with her day-to-day functioning. In fact, according to one study, GAD was associated with more lost workdays than any other condition, including asthma, hypertension, diabetes, arthritis, and Major Depression.

Female gender is a risk factor for GAD; the lifetime risk is 3.6 percent in men, 6.6 percent in women. This difference holds true across cultures as diverse as Brazil and Turkey. The difference emerges early in life; at age six, girls already have a twofold risk compared with boys.

One wonders whether various psychosocial aspects of girls' development might account for this disparity. And indeed, several factors have been shown to increase girls' risk of developing GAD: self-consciousness, lower self-esteem, physical illness, to name a few. But even controlling for these variables, girls remain at higher risk, suggesting a biologic basis.

Data from epidemiological studies show that, in addition to gender, several psychosocial factors are associated with GAD. In particular, ethnic-minority status and low socioeconomic status are correlated with high rates of GAD. Among African American women, the incidence may be as high as 10 percent.

Panic Disorder

Mrs. D. is a woman in her forties, married, a secretary in the insurance office of a local hospital. She is brought by her husband to the emergency room because of the abrupt onset of difficulty breathing, palpitations, chest pain, and a panicky feeling that she is "going to die." Her husband says that these symptoms came on "out of the blue," just as the family was sitting down to dinner. She has not been sick, nor has she lately seemed anxious or depressed. On examination, her heart rate is rapid, her blood pressure slightly elevated, but otherwise her exam and electrocardiogram are normal.

The hallmark of Panic Disorder is the panic attack. As in the case described here, panic attacks are defined as the abrupt onset of an acutely distressing physical state: palpitations or racing heartbeat, shortness of breath, dizziness, tingling sensations in the hands, nausea, or dizziness. This very physical experience is accompanied by an intense subjective feeling of anxiety or fear; usually, a fear of dying, losing control, or "going crazy." Panic attacks are very discrete events, occurring over several minutes; they may be preceded by a fear-provoking stimulus, such as an exam or job interview, or they may seem to arise spontaneously. Spontaneous panic attacks are perceived as "coming out of the blue," under entirely normal, nonstressful circumstances. To constitute full-blown Panic Disorder, two or more spontaneous panic attacks must have occurred.

Panic Disorder is often, though not inevitably, accompanied by agoraphobia: this likelihood is higher in women than in men. *Agoraphobia* means, literally, fear of the marketplace. The moniker is interesting in itself, suggesting on the one hand, a phobic avoidance of the public places in which women have traditionally been found; and, on the other, a reluctance to enter the more modern "markets"—for instance, businesses, professional institutions—inhabited by men. In the most extreme cases, agoraphobics are confined to their homes for months or even years; those less severely afflicted leave the home but tend to avoid public places, such as buses, trains, and bridges, from which rapid escape would be impossible.

Panic Disorder, like GAD, is twice as common among women than men (2.3 percent versus 1.0 percent incidence). As with GAD, too, this difference holds true across cultures. In a recent study, rates of Panic Disorder were similar in African American, Hispanic, and white groups, although the rate of agoraphobia was higher among African Americans.

Perhaps because panic attacks are defined by relatively discrete, reproducible physiologic symptoms, they have been extensively studied from a biological perspective. Multiple neurotransmitter systems have been implicated, including serotonin, norepinephrine, and gamma-aminobutyric acid (GABA), the neurotransmitter that induces relaxation and sleep. These neurotransmitters may exert their effects by interfering with the body's internal stress-regulation system. . . .

More recently, researchers have postulated a link between biologic and psychosocial precipitants of Panic Disorder. They suggest that a propensity to anxiety may be linked to early parental loss or separation, leading to subsequent problems with attachment. In this model, children with an underlying predisposition to anxiety might suffer a disruption in the parental relationship, leading to a heightened response to future separations or losses.

Social Phobia

Ms. M. is a twenty-five-year-old graduate student in music who presents to her school clinic for help with longstanding social fears. She does well in her assignments, but is so anxious in class that she cannot ask or answer a question. She avoids socializing at school and spends most of her time at home reading or studying. As a child, she was extremely shy and had difficulty transitioning to school. She would like to have friends, but each time she approaches someone to talk, she panics.

The fear of humiliating oneself in public is so ubiquitous that labeling it a disorder might seem inapt. Like a propensity to worry, shyness and self-consciousness are character traits that afflict many, if not most, of us at one time or another. In fact, community studies show that roughly one-third of all people consider themselves to be more anxious than other people in social situations. Such anxiety only crosses the threshold for Social Phobia when it becomes persistent, irrational, and interferes with daily functioning.

The defining feature of Social Phobia is an intense fear of social situations in which a person might act in a humiliating manner. People with Social Phobia tend to avoid public encounters, such as parties, interviews, and restaurants, or to endure them only with great difficulty. They also recognize that their anxiety is out of proportion to the actual situation. Common themes in Social Phobia include fears about meeting new people, making oral presentations, using a public restroom, writing, talking or eating in public.

Social Phobia is often complicated by other conditions, such as depression, Panic Disorder, and agoraphobia. Because these conditions also contribute to social withdrawal (and because sufferers are loathe to come to treatment), Social Phobia can be difficult to diagnose. A key factor is that people with Social Phobia are afraid to interact with *people*, whereas those with agoraphobia are afraid of *environments* or situations from which they cannot easily escape.

The rate of Social Phobia has been variably reported. More recent estimates have placed the lifetime prevalence at 13.3 percent, making it the third most common psychological disorder, after Major Depression (17.1 percent) and alcohol dependence (14.1 percent). Women are more often affected than men, with a ratio of 3:2. Interestingly, although women are more likely to have Social Phobia, men are more likely to seek treatment. Some researchers have attributed this discrepancy to gender role typing; they argue that men have traditionally been expected to be more confident and outgoing in social situations than women, therefore reticence would for them cause more impairment and, possibly, more subjective distress. Data from some studies of natural shyness support this theory; shy boys are more likely to suffer social and occupational dysfunction as adults than are shy girls. . . .

Comorbidity and Outcome

Most anxiety disorders have a persistent, chronic course. Without treatment roughly two-thirds of affected persons will remain symptomatic at five-year follow-up. Additionally, anxiety disorders tend to coexist, both with one another and with a host of other conditions. Major Depression, substance abuse, and eating disorders are often comorbid with anxiety.

The Impact of Stress on Women

BraVada Garrett-Akinsanya

Stress and its impact on physical and mental health often makes headlines in the fast-paced, technologically driven world of the twenty-first century. Multitasking has become an expected part of life for most women who are trying to juggle children, spouses, household duties, and workplace responsibilities. In the following selection BraVada Garrett-Akinsanya discusses the positive and negative effects of stress and the unique factors that make women more likely to feel the pressures of stress than men. Stress can be a good aspect of a woman's life because it can help her stay motivated to reach her goals, Garrett-Akinsanya notes, but it can also have a negative impact that may lead to exhaustion, immunological impairment, and psychological disorders. Garrett-Akinsanya asserts that a number of stress factors are unique to women, including women's traditional roles as family caretakers and the lack of power in social relationships. In addition, while all women are more susceptible to stress-induced illness, minority women are even more likely to suffer from stress-related hypertension and heart disease. Ultimately, stress can become disabling to women because they are more likely to continue struggling than ask for help. Garrett-Akinsanya is a licensed psychologist and president of Brakins Consulting and Psychological Services.

Women have a unique familiarity with stress. For many women, stress begins before they get out of bed. Imagine for a moment being awakened from a deep (and well-deserved) sleep by a four-year-old wanting breakfast. You get

BraVada Garrett-Akinsanya, "Stress Management for Women," *The Complete Guide to Mental Health for Women*, edited by Lauren Slater, Jessica Henderson Daniel, and Amy Elizabeth Banks. Boston: Beacon Press, 2003. Copyright © 2003 by Beacon Press. All rights reserved. Reproduced by permission.

up (while your partner—if you have one—is still sleeping) and go to the kitchen to prepare breakfast and pack lunches for your family. By now, it's time to get everyone dressed for the day, and you are challenged with everything from looking for your child's lost sneakers to assisting your partner with selecting a clothes ensemble. Before you go to work, you probably have the responsibility of dropping off the kids, checking homework before the bus comes, and maybe even taking out the garbage. By the time you go to the office for the 8:30 A. M. meeting with an important client, you're exhausted!

While the presence of life stress for many women is a commonly shared experience, knowledge about the positive and negative components of stress often eludes us. Some basic knowledge about stress will lead you to a conceptual understanding of its positive and negative components. The rationale here is that if we, as women, understand ourselves and stress processes better, perhaps we can apply that knowledge to creating healthier, more productive choices for ourselves.

What Is Stress?

First, our discussion of stress must begin with a definition of what stress is and what it is not. There is also a need to discriminate between stress, stressors, stress reactions, and strain. *Stress* is the general concept of describing an internal or external "load" on the human system. A *stressor*, then, is a specifie issue or challenge (external or internal) from which the "load" is derived. A *stress reaction* is the individual's reaction to a given stressor (whether it is physiological, behavioral, emotional, or cognitive). Furthermore, a stress reaction may be described as a responsive state of arousal that is characterized by physiological, emotional, and cognitive/perceptual components.

Within this context, experiencing stress is not solely a "bad" thing. Surely, it beats the alternative: a lack of arousal—or death! Consequently, the presence of a certain amount of stress is necessary and fulfills a basic human need for arousal and stimulation. Key studies in psychology have linked the need for arousal and stimulation to infant depression/death and brain development as well as to motivational factors in adults. Thus, when stress occurs within the context of the ordinary human arousal necessary to accomplish daily activities, it is a "good" thing. The presence of stress is even better when it serves a motivational function and creates within us a positive, exhilarating, and challenging experience that can lead to higher levels of performance. This level of increased performance caused by motivational stress is known as "eustress."

Strain, on the other hand, is the prolonged impact of the stressor on the system that can create overload, fatigue, and precursors to illness. Generally, when people refer to stress they are really talking about strain or "stress overload." Stress overload is a serious problem. Some reports have suggested that between 75 and 90 percent of all visits to primary care physicians are for stress-related complaints or disorders. Stress overload has been linked to many of the leading causes of death such as heart disease, cancer, lung ailments, accidents, cirrhosis, and suicide. It is also estimated 1 million workers are absent on an average workday because of stress-related complaints. Finally, a three-year study conducted by a large corporation showed that 60 percent of employee absences were due to psychological problems such as stress overload.

Consequently, it is the circumstance of experiencing stress overload that can lead to conditions of inadequate levels of functioning known as "distress." Most women can readily identify states of distress because they are often preceded by incidents of failure, threat, embarrassment, disappointment, and other negative experiences.

What Are Some Signs and Symptoms of Stress Overload?

Each woman not only has a unique vulnerability to stress responses, but each person also has a unique and specific way in which she responds to stress. Each woman may exhibit unique symptoms and vulnerabilities in reactions to stress depending on factors such as her unique biological makeup, genetics, environmental situations, social support, and even the way she goes about making an interpretation of circumstances (whether she tends to be an optimist or a pessimist). Consequently, the signs of stress may vary among individuals to include symptoms that are physiological, emotional, or cognitive/perceptual in nature.

Physiological Signs and Symptoms of Stress The physical symptoms of stress are first experienced through a gland called the hypothalamus, which produces at least nine different hormones as that communicate to other glands in your body either a need for arousal or rest. These systems work together to orchestrate a heightened state of arousal as a physiological reaction to stress and are your body's way of getting you prepared for a "flight-or-fight" experience that is designed to preserve life. Studies have shown that women who are chronically exposed to daily experiences of the physical symptoms of stress (anxiety, racing heartbeat, digestive problems, increased blood flow, tensed muscles, elevated levels of hormones), run greater risks of experiencing health problems, particularly infection risk and hypertension.

Some of the key physical signs and symptoms of stress include, but are not limited to, increased heart rate, elevated blood pressure, sweaty palms, tightness of the chest, neck, jaws, and back muscles. Other physiological symptoms include headaches, diarrhea, constipation, difficulty urinating, trembling, twitching, stuttering, and speech difficulties. Finally, some women complain that when they experience stress, they have symptoms of nausea, vomiting, sleep disturbances/ insomnia, changes in eating habits, fatigue, shallow breathing, dryness of the mouth or throat, cold hands, itching, and chronic pain.

Emotional Signs and Symptoms of Stress While some women report that they experience emotional signs and symptoms of stress such as irritability, outbursts of anger, hostility, and depression, others report symptoms such as increased jealousy, restlessness, withdrawal, anxiousness, diminished initiative, feelings of unreality or overalertness, reduction of personal involvement with others, and lack of interest in previously enjoyable activities. Finally, some women describe that they experience emotional symptoms of stress that include an increased tendency to cry, being critical of others, self-deprecation, nightmares, impatience, decreased perception of positive outcomes, narrowed focus, obsessive rumination, reduced self-esteem, and less positive reactions to events.

Women who are placed in conditions of prolonged, insidious stress (such as conditions associated with sexual discrimination, unemployment, violence/abuse, harassment, etc., in the workplace) may report experiencing symptoms of what is known as the General Adaptation Syndrome (GAS). Women who experience the GAS have also experienced prolonged periods of overexposure to arousal/stress, followed by a period of resistance and a period that is finally concluded by an experience of "exhaustion." A woman who reaches the exhaustion or "burnout" phase may feel that she has been emotionally drained or beaten and may also feel that she must "give up." Her emotional reaction of "letting go," "fleeing," or "giving up" may involve characteristics of "survivors guilt" because she may perceive that her choice to either abandon a cause or become physically removed from the environment leaves other women (potential victims) vulnerable.

Cognitive Perceptual Signs and Symptoms of Stress The cognitive/perceptual signs and symptoms of stress are usually the ones that may be first noticed by others. These symptoms include forgetfulness, blocking, blurred vision, errors in judging distance, diminished or exaggerated fantasy life, as well as reduced reactivity, productivity, and concentration. Other symptoms of cognitive/perceptual disturbances include a lack of attention to detail, a preoccupation with or orientation to the past, and decreased psychomotor reactivity and coordination. Some women report attention deficits, disorganization of thought, negative self-esteem, a decrease of meaning in life, as well as a negative evaluation of themselves, the future, and the situation. Finally, some women may notice that when they are under stress they perceive that they lack control or have a need for too much control.

When stress reaches the level at which it negatively impacts a woman's ability to attend to details or concentrate, her risks of under-performing or getting into accidents are increased. Some statistics state that 60 to 80 percent of work-related accidents are due to stress.

What Are Some Stress Factors Unique to Women?

Women experience some stress-related factors that appear to be more prevalent among them. For example, women tend to be more vulnerable to stress-induced illnesses, and their vulnerability can be traced back not only to familial biology and genetic predispositions, but also to women's socialization. From early childhood, girls are socialized to inevitably take on the roles and responsibilities of caretakers. Additionally, because of power differentials in terms of gender, women are often not well positioned in relationships (whether work-related or personal) to have as much control of their environment as men have. One researcher has examined the stressful nature of gender stereotypes and its impact on the task performance among females. This concept, known as *stereotyped threat*, implies that if we think that people hold unfair or unrealistic expectations of us, we may experience levels of stress that detract from (rather than motivate) our ability to perform optimally.

For women of diverse sexual orientations, ethnicity, or immigrant status, the challenges are even greater. Studies have shown that women of minority groups are at even greater risks for stress-related health problems such as hypertension or other types of cardiovascular diseases. Several studies have demonstrated that risk factors are compounded among these groups because of the multiple social, physical, and economic disparities that exist for women of color in terms of access to resources and services when needed. One study among women who were overextended looked at coping strategies in which women were given a choice of seeking support, letting some tasks go, or working harder. The study revealed that the majority of the women chose to "work harder" rather than to ask for help or to let things go.

Some Causes of Eating Disorders in Women

Deborah Marcontell Michel and Susan G. Willard

Recent reports indicate that cases of eating disorders, especially among young girls and women, are increasing at alarming rates. In an attempt to understand why some females develop eating disorders but others do not, Deborah Marcontell Michel and Susan G. Willard explore the biological, psychological, and sociological reasons behind the development of anorexia and bulimia. In the following selection Michel and Willard clearly point out the complexities of the disorders and that no single factor solely contributes to their development. Genetic and psychological history, societal influences such as images of women's bodies in the media, individual personality characteristics, and family dynamics combine to form a powerful mixture that impacts thousands of young girls and women each year. Michel and Willard are professors in the department of psychiatry and neurology at the Tulane University School of Medicine. In addition, Willard is the director of the Eating Disorders Treatment Center at River Oaks Hospital in New Orleans.

No one knows exactly how or why an eating disorder occurs. We do know that there is no single reason for someone to develop one of these illnesses, and we know that eating disorders are not about food. The thoughts and behaviors having to do with eating, weight, and body image are symptoms of deeper psychological conflicts and issues that drive the eating disordered behavior. Just as fever signals some sort of infection that a person's body is trying to fight, an eating disorder is indicative of other underlying problems. The fact

Deborah Marcontell Michel and Susan G. Willard, *When Dieting Becomes Dangerous: A Guide to Understanding and Treating Anorexia and Bulimia.* New Haven, CT: Yale University Press, 2003. Copyright © 2003 by Deborah Marcontell Michel and Susan G. Willard. All rights reserved. Reproduced by permission.

that the principal concerns of eating disorders are not actually food, calories, and weight often confuses families and friends because food and weight related issues are the obvious focus of the eating disordered individual. For example, the anorexic will adamantly complain that she is fat and must restrict calories to lose more weight. The bulimic may claim that vomiting is the only way she can control her weight. Both often say that if it were not for problems with food and weight, they would be fine. . . .

Biological Factors

A great deal of the research examining biological factors that may make some young women more susceptible to eating disorders has focused on genetic components. In particular, researchers have compared the prevalence of anorexia in sets of identical and fraternal twins. Difficulties with this type of research include the small sample sizes, how patients are recruited for studies, differences in the definitions of anorexia, the extent to which twins share a similar environment, and similarities in social life (environmental factors). In any case, researchers who have reviewed studies with satisfactory designs report that there is evidence of a genetic predisposition to anorexia. Unknown, however, is the degree to which genetics influences the development of the disorder. What may actually be "inherited" are certain personality characteristics or traits that increase susceptibility to the development of an eating disorder. In particular, those with anxious, obsessional, and perfectionistic personality traits seem more vulnerable. Additionally, studies have shown that a high percentage of women with anorexia, up to 90 percent in one study, had an anxiety disorder before the onset of anorexia. This finding, again, suggests that excessive anxiety may be a risk factor for anorexia. . . .

Although binge eating is primarily psychologically motivated, a biological vulnerability may be due in part to the body's attempts to compensate for the effects of rigorous dieting and physiological food deprivation. More specifically, girls and women who starve themselves or chronically diet may be trying to maintain a weight below that which is natural and healthy for body frame and height. Those who attempt to maintain an unhealthy weight may experience biologically driven eating behavior (such as binge eating) that is aimed at increasing weight to the body's preferred status. This kind of biologically driven binge eating has been observed in other groups subjected to starvation or chronic food restriction, such as prisoners of war or laboratory subjects who did not have eating disorders. . . .

Societal Influences

There are numerous ways in which our society contributes to the obsession of girls and women with beauty, fitness, and—most important—thinness. Our culture has spawned an atmosphere in which females feel pressured to be successful by society's unrealistic standards to be "superwoman." Standards for success include being thin and beautiful, having husbands and children, and pursuing professions and careers that carry with them power and financial prowess. Confusion, anxiety, and concern about these role expectations, and ambivalence about one's position in society, are thought to be related to the increase in eating disorders seen in our culture and around the world. These disturbing feelings may propel some girls and women to look to their appearance as a way to feel in control. Today's greater sexual freedom for women is a phenomenon that produces even more anxiety and fear. The end result is a physical obsession of epidemic proportions, wherein up to 80 percent of teenage girls worry about being overweight and children as young as five years of age have body image concerns and fear becoming overweight. Unhealthy dieting is extremely common in girls and women who believe that losing weight and perfecting their bodies is the answer to life's problems. . . .

It is virtually impossible these days to browse through a magazine, read a newspaper, or watch television for any substantial period without seeing the promotion of diets, exercise programs, fitness centers, and/or dietary aids. This media hype has led to the popularity of dieting among young women and adolescent girls, with 75 percent of female teenagers dieting before the age of sixteen. Furthermore, the last two decades have seen an increase in the use of dietary aids such as diet pills, exercise equipment, and materials designed to teach people how to lose weight. The 1990s saw an explosion in the number of specific diets and diet books on the market. In fact, it was recently estimated that Americans spend about $40 billion per year in pursuit of thinness!

It should be obvious at this point that we are a culture preoccupied with body shape and weight, and that our values of beauty relate disproportionately to thinness. The real danger, however, lies in the fact that this overvaluation of beauty and thinness often leads to early and stringent dieting, which has been shown to be the most common factor leading to the development of eating disorders. . . .

Women who actively attempt to meet the current ideal of thinness and do not take into consideration personal body frame and/or natural weight setpoint (that is, biologically favored weight), may find it not only psychologically frustrating to lose weight, but biologically difficult or impossible. The issue is further complicated by the finding that healthy Caucasian women are apt to overestimate their actual body size. This tendency is commonly referred to as distorted body image. Not surprisingly, it is almost always present in eating disordered individuals. Ironically, even if someone with an eating disorder attains what she deems to be the social ideal of thinness, she is unlikely to acknowledge that she is thin enough because of her distorted body image. In other words, she is likely to continue to see herself as fat, even after significant weight loss. With the popularity of plastic surgery, particularly liposuction, such misperceptions about the body are leading to pathological and repetitive requests for surgery that may represent a modified version of purging behavior. . . .

Individual Personality Characteristics

Most girls and young women in our culture are subjected to societal pressures for thinness that may lead them to diet, but not all of them develop eating disorders. Along with societal pressures and biological factors that may contribute to the development of eating disorders, certain personality characteristics have been linked to women who develop these illnesses. Low self-esteem and perfectionism as well as the need for achievement, control, and approval are traits consistently seen in such individuals.

Anorexics tend to be quite anxious; they strive to please everyone around them and avoid any source of potential conflict. When young, anorexics tend to be "model children" who are always compliant and rarely display normal teenage rebellion. These characteristics ultimately prevent them from recognizing and honestly expressing their feelings. Fears of sexuality and a refusal to grow up are commonly seen. Arthur Crisp, an international expert on anorexia, has described it as "an abortion of development" and a "maturational crisis."

Bulimics may have any combination of the features listed above, though on average they tend to show more emotionality than those with anorexia. They are more likely, for instance, to experience intense emotions that are confusing to them, such as alternating among feelings of happiness, despair, and anger. Often they are not sure why they feel as they do. Bulimics are more likely to exhibit teenage rebellion seen in self-destructive behaviors such as alcohol or other drug abuse, sexual promiscuity, or shoplifting.

An important emotional feature that stems in part from the characteristics already mentioned is lack of identity. When an individual is unable to figure out what she feels, why she feels as she does, or how to have her emotional needs met in a healthy manner, it is difficult for her to form a sense of self. When she is busy living up to the expectations of others and trying to please those around her, she is prevented from discovering her own values and opinions as well as what she really desires for herself. . . .

[Such aforementioned] personality traits . . . can inhibit formation of identity and result in inadequate or faulty coping skills, preventing young women from effectively dealing with life's stresses and problems. In addition, these characteristics often increase the vulnerability of young women to cultural pressures for thinness in their attempts to be perfect or at least to improve themselves. They may then turn to their bodies as an imagined means of coping with the problems in their lives and as a way to feel in control.

Family Characteristics

There are women affected by societal pressures for thinness who diet and possess the [previously mentioned] personality characteristics . . . , but do not succumb to eating disorders. What, then, might be another ingredient that contributes to the development of an eating disorder?

Although no one knows for sure what role the family plays in this context, we do know that the family provides the backdrop against which eating disorders develop. For decades, clinicians have noted the association between eating disorders and difficulty with individuation and emotional separation from the family of origin. Individuation refers to a person's ability to establish a separate identity, including opinions, tastes, values, and goals that differ from those of the family of origin. In those who successfully complete this necessary developmental task, an overlap may remain among opinions, values, and goals, yet an independent and distinct sense of self emerges, which differs from that of the family. Family therapists have frequently described families who have a daughter with an eating disorder as enmeshed (emotionally overinvolved with fused identities), making separation difficult.

It is never useful or appropriate to blame any family member or members for the development of an eating disorder; these illnesses are complex and occur for a variety of reasons. However, as we know that the family represents the holding environment for the child, it is always important to look at which aspects of the family might relate to occurrence of the disease. . . .

One common system is the "perfect family," in which rigid rules consciously or unconsciously govern the behavior of all family members. The female with an eating disorder in this type of family tends to be a very high achiever by family standards. The family reputation is sacred; the members are expected to think, act, and feel the "right" way. Appearance is of utmost importance, as this family type needs to seem "perfect" to outside observers. An eating disorder in this family system may help the anorexic or bulimic to accomplish one or more of the following: (1) passive rebellion against the family system; (2) creation of a separate identity; (3) suppression of feelings by focusing on food; and (4) assertion of control over herself in the midst of a controlling family.

A second family type is the "overprotective family," characterized by its nurturance of dependence and refusal to acknowledge any need for independence. Anger and conflict are not well tolerated and are seldom overtly displayed. Since the adolescent period is fraught with change and conflict, many difficult issues are never openly or directly resolved. As a result, passive-aggressive behaviors develop, thereby hindering direct expressions of rebellion. Eating disorder symptoms in this family type may serve as a means of passively rebelling against the family and indirectly expressing anger, while simultaneously reaffirming dependence on the family members. In this way, the eating disordered family member does not risk direct anger, criticism, or rejection by the rest of the family because she is viewed as "sick." . . .

Certain other family characteristics are commonly found among families with an eating disordered child. Often another family member is either overweight or excessively thin. There may be an overconcern with food and food-related issues in the household. It is not unusual to see one or both parents involved with chronic dieting and/or rigid exercise regimens. Daughters of these families may be particularly susceptible to dieting and exercising as a means of bonding with parents who are obviously preoccupied with such matters themselves.

Some parents of children with eating disorders live their lives vicariously through their children and their children's successes and accomplishments. When these youngsters start to show signs of puberty or adolescence, the parents often get depressed or frightened about what the future will hold when the children are fully grown and gone. The unconscious pressure on these children is to stay young and not grow up. Family loyalty to maintaining the status quo is often chosen over normal development, which would lead to separation and independence.

Other characteristics that may be present in some form include a critical parent, one or more parents with depression, and/or the presence of marital problems (which may give the child the spoken or unspoken message that if she grows up and becomes independent, the family system will fall apart).

Black Women's Mental Health Needs Go Unmet

Shauna Curphey

While it is estimated that 60 percent of African American women suffer from depression, few of them pursue professional treatment for their illnesses. In the following selection Shauna Curphey argues that this resistance to seeking help is the result of cultural stigmas and lack of professionals who specialize in African American mental health issues. Recent studies have revealed the close relationship between mental and physical health. These studies maintain that women suffering from serious mental health problems have a harder time living with and healing from chronic illnesses. Given that African American women are more likely than other women to suffer from heart disease, stroke, and high blood pressure, Curphey states that treating their mental health problems is of utmost importance to their well-being. Curphey is currently a law student whose writing has appeared in several publications, including Progressive Woman *and* Washington Law and Politics.

"There's a fear of putting our business in the street . . . of somehow revealing too much," said Latonya Slack, executive director of the California Black Women's Health Project, an Inglewood, Calif., community-health organization. "Black women can perceive going to a therapist as something we don't do," she added.

Lorraine Cole, president of the Black Women's Health Imperative, the Washington, D.C.-based parent organization of the California Black Women's Health Project, agrees. "There's a deep-seated feeling that going to seek professional help is a sign of weakness," she said.

In California, African American women have the shortest life expectancy among women of all racial and ethnic groups in the state. They also have the highest mortality rate for heart disease and stroke and the highest prevalence of high blood pressure and obesity. Recent research indicates that mental health plays a role in these health disparities in California—and across the nation. But while many black women know and discuss the threats to their physical health, when it comes to mental health, there's silence and inaction.

Slack and Cole, both African American women, are leading efforts to address the physical, mental and spiritual health needs of black women. Both have commissioned studies that revealed many black women are struggling with mental health issues but are not seeking professional help. They and others see improving black women's access to mental health treatment as a crucial element to addressing the serious, but often manageable, illnesses plaguing their physical health.

Women Who Need Care Go Without

Despite the emotional and physical consequences of mental-health problems, black women are less likely to seek treatment. The percentage of African Americans overall who receive needed mental-health care is only half that of whites, according to a 2001 Surgeon General report on mental health. By some estimates, only 7 percent of black women suffering from depression receive any treatment, compared with 20 percent of the general population.

Last year, Slack's organization, the California Black Women's Health Project, released the results of a study of more than 1,300 African American women across the state. The subjects in the study revealed that they tended to repress feelings, let frustration build and release tension through tears or conflict. The findings of the study, which included a series of focus group discussions across the state, led Slack to launch a mental health initiative to improve African American women's acceptance of and access to mental health treatment.

The California Black Women's Health Project launched several programs to address the disparities in black women's mental health in the state. In August 2002, the project began hosting town hall meetings that bring together black women, mental health providers and state and local policy makers to discuss black women's health concerns. They have held four meetings in Southern California and started outreach in the northern part of the state with a town hall meeting in Oakland last weekend.

Through the course of these meetings and their annual policy summit, held in Sacramento in February, the organization has developed the 12 Commandments of Mental Health, a secular self-help tool for African American women. Still in draft form, the list of guidelines includes "Self care is not selfish—take care of you so you can take care of others," and "Recognize something is wrong—you deserve to feel well." "We're working on getting women to accept mental and emotional well-being as their birthright," said Slack.

New 'Commandments' for Use in Churches

Since the California study revealed that more than 90 percent of black women believe their spiritual and religious beliefs affect their health, Slack plans to use the 12 Commandments in an outreach program with local churches. She recently submitted a proposal to the California Department of Health to organize a group of licensed mental health providers who would commit to partner with and serve faith-based institutions and their members.

The California Black Women's Health Project is also working with state lawmakers to create a student-loan-forgiveness program for licensed mental health providers who serve low-income communities of color. In addition, the project is advocating a voluntary cultural-competency certification program for licensed mental health providers. The certification would prove that providers had completed training in how to recognize and respond to the cultural differences among their patients.

These programs could serve as a model for national efforts to address black women's mental health needs, said Cole.

Gloria Morrow is a licensed clinical psychologist in Pomona, Calif., with a private practice in which 90 percent of the patients are African American women. Having heard the collective grief, pain and worry of her patients, she said these efforts to highlight their mental-health needs are crucial because "there's nothing worse than suffering in silence." She says that, for many of her patients, racism and sexism play out in the workplace, in their relationships with men and often lead to low self-esteem, depression and anxiety.

"This whole notion that racism is dead is a falsehood because people continue to suffer," Morrow said.

Morrow said that the distrust and stigma that black women feel about mental-health treatment, in her view, arise in part from their difficulty in finding a therapist to whom they can readily relate. African Americans comprise less than 2 percent of licensed psychiatrists in California and less than 4 percent of mental-health care providers nationally. Overcoming this shortage may be crucial to improving treatment outcomes for African American women. In her work as a consultant for a local mental health facility, Morrow has so far found from interviews with clients that mental-health practitioners "don't get it when they are working with people who don't look like them."

Pursuing Perfection Amid Criticism, Doubts

In the California study conducted by the California Black Women's Health Project, one focus group participant described the pressure she felt juggling school and work while dealing with society's negative perception of black men as she tries to raise her son. Another described the racism she encounters at her bank job, where she is the only black employee and where she feels white customers frequently treat her as if she doesn't know what she is talking about. Overall, the focus group discussions revealed that black women are overwhelmed by the pursuit of perfectionism, meeting goals, mediating family conflicts and challenging the criticisms and doubts of others.

Racism and Domestic Violence

Racism also feeds the violence experienced by black women, as the internalized rage of African American men against their mistreatment may manifest itself in anger and violence toward women, according to the 2002 Women of Color Health Data Book, a report released by the U.S. Department of Health and Human Services. More than one-third of black women in California have been victims of physical violence and more than one half have been victims of verbal abuse, according to the California Black Women's Health Project study.

Nationally, 43 percent of black women report they were verbally or emotionally abused while growing up. Approximately 20 percent reported they were physically abused as a child and another 22 percent said they were sexually abused, according to a 2001 study conducted for the Black Women's Health Imperative. In the California study, a majority of survey respondents said violence has had an impact on their health.

Economic Insecurity

Besides racism and violence, African American women also struggle with economic insecurity. The poverty rate for black women is 25 percent, more than twice the rate among white women, according to the latest statistics from the U.S. Census Bureau. In addition, 43 percent of black families are maintained by women with no spouse present. The stress of trying to make ends meet may translate directly into the finding that

African Americans living below the poverty level have the highest rate of depression for any racial or ethnic group, according to research cited by the Women of Color Health Data Book.

But mental health problems are not confined to low-income women. African American women higher on the socioeconomic ladder experience their own set of pressures, especially in the workplace, where they feel they are often treated as if they do not deserve to be there, said Morrow. As a result, black women struggle with a pressure to out-perform others just to gain acceptance. She used her own career as an example.

"I had to be at the top of my class," said Morrow in a phone interview, "I was always seeing myself being compared and competing with this white ghost . . . These issues play out in the lives of black folk. It is impacting how they feel about themselves and it is impacting their physical and mental health."

Sixty percent of African American women have symptoms of depression, according to the national study conducted for the Black Women's Health Imperative. In addition, research indicates that the stress in the lives of African American women contributes to poor physical health. Stress related to racism may underlie the poor diet and resulting obesity among black women and may be associated with the high prevalence of high blood pressure and diabetes, according to the Women of Color Health Data Book.

Lack of insurance also contributes to the low percentage of black women who seek mental health treatment. Nearly one in four African Americans is uninsured. Even among those who have coverage, mental health may not be included in the policy or the cap on covered expenses may be low. But better insurance coverage alone is not enough to get more women to seek help. African American women also struggle against the stigma associated with mental-health treatment.

Fear of Treatment

One study found that the proportion of African Americans who feared mental-health treatment was more than twice that of whites, according to the surgeon general's report. Part of the fear stems from wariness of the medical establishment that arises from past abuses, said Slack, such as the Tuskegee experiment. (In 1932, the federal government sponsored a study to examine the impact of untreated syphilis involving black men. The experiment went on until 1972 without the test subjects' knowledge and most of the subjects died without receiving treatment.) As a result of the distrust engendered by the now-infamous experiment and the stigma associated with seeking help, many black women rely on spiritual leaders and community members to handle personal problems. There's also an added pressure from the ethic of the strong black woman, a cultural value that promotes toughness and self-sacrifice.

"There are so many women who are not diagnosed or are under-diagnosed who are just existing on a thread," Slack concluded. ". . . They think 'My mother suffered. My grandmother suffered. It's just the lot of black women in America.' It doesn't have to be that way."

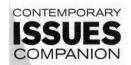

CHAPTER 4

Personal Narratives
on Women's Health

My Mother Gave Me Anorexia

"Juliette Potter," as told to Stacy Colino

In the following selection Juliette Potter (not her real name) describes how her mother's obsession with her weight led Juliette to
develop anorexia. Juliette explains that her mother, who herself
suffers from disordered eating behaviors, began to limit Juliette's
food intake when she was only four years old. As Juliette gained
the weight that was normal for a growing child, her worried
mother would organize contests to see which one of them could
lose the most pounds. By the time Juliette was a junior in high
school, she had developed full-blown anorexia. Juliette states
that, with therapy and hospitalization, she has started normalizing her relationship with food. However, Juliette confides, she has
found that she must keep her distance from her mother because
of her unhealthy influence. Stacy Colino has written for Cosmo-
politan, Parents, and Working Mother.

For as long as I can remember, my mother focused on my
weight. I was never heavy as a kid, but I had a big appetite
and a little bit of a belly, and that worried her intensely. By
the time I was 4, my mom had already replaced my apple
juice with Diet Coke, and I continued to diet throughout my
childhood. Whenever I lost weight, she would get really excited and literally dance around. Later on, I realized that my
mother's way of thinking was twisted, but by then, it was too
late: I had developed a deadly eating disorder.

A Mother's Influence

I grew up as an only child in a somewhat unsettled household. My parents divorced when I was 9, and I went back and
forth between their homes every week. My mother and I were

more like friends than mother and daughter, but she was still a big influence on me—and her own eating habits were very unhealthy. Her favorite diet was one where she wouldn't eat all day, then for one hour at night, she could eat whatever she wanted as long as it was within that hour. As she struggled with her own cravings, my mom tried to limit my food intake as well. If we went out for a pizza and I reached for a second slice she'd say, "Don't you think you've had enough?" I was a growing kid, and when my pajamas would get too small, she'd warn me that I had to eat less.

Soon, I figured out my own ways to curb my appetite. In fifth grade, I bought diet pills at the drugstore and took them for about a month. Sometimes, when I wanted to lose weight, I would go for a week eating nothing but bagels. As I got older, I started developing different food rules—for example, I could have pizza after school only on the days that I also had gymnastics because then I could work off the calories. My mom and I would go grocery shopping together, and we'd stock up on low-fat foods like pretzels, tuna, and frozen yogurt. There was no letup, not even on our vacations to Club Med, where my mom would orchestrate a contest of who could lose the most weight while we were there.

During the summer of 1997, I turned 16 and spent a month taking an SAT prep course at the University of California in Los Angeles (UCLA). By that point, my eating habits had become very strange—I'd concoct weird combinations like pickles and ketchup or sandwiches with just sprouts and honey mustard and while I was there, I lost about 10 pounds. When I flew home and got off the plane, the first thing my mom said was "Oh, my God! You look great!" Then she took me shopping for a whole new wardrobe. I had begun my steep descent into anorexia.

Spiraling Out of Control

By the fall of my junior year, I was counting calories more and eating much less. I'd have coffee or tea in the morning and I wouldn't eat all day, but I'd drink lots of water. Then, at eight o'clock at night, I'd have frozen spinach, cooked in the microwave, with ketchup. I was eating 150 to 300 calories a day—my max was 500—and that was counting gum and hard candies. At a certain point, a switch went off in my brain, and I didn't have any control over what I was doing.

In three and a half months, I lost 20 pounds. My weight dropped down to 91 pounds—at 5 feet 5 inches and with my build, I should have weighed around 125. I was out of it and confused all the time. I also stopped getting my period. But I felt proud of how thin I was and was shocked at other people's negative reactions. One time, I wore overalls to school, and everyone acted really funny around me. Apparently, the pants were so baggy that I looked skeletal, but I just couldn't see it at the time.

Neither could my mother. My boyfriend called her several times, begging her to take me to a doctor. Finally, she took me to my pediatrician, who said "Sometimes, teenagers get sad" and told my mom I was fine. But after seeing me one weekend, my dad stepped in and made me go to a doctor who specializes in eating disorders. My mom came with me, and when the doctor told her I weighed 91 pounds, she started crying. It was as if she needed a concrete number to finally realize that something was really wrong with me.

Dealing with the Problem

The doctor said I needed to be hospitalized, so in December 1997, I was pulled out of high school and spent a month in an adolescent-medicine unit on Long Island. It was basically a refeeding program, although there were also therapy sessions about body image. Every morning, I had to step on a scale. If I lost any weight, I'd have to wear a hospital gown all day. If I didn't finish a meal, I'd have to drink an Ensure, a meal-replacement drink. If I didn't do that, I'd get a feeding tube up my nose. I felt controlled and caged, but inevitably, I started gaining weight. After my hospital stay, I was in day treatment for another six weeks, so I didn't go back to school until February 1998.

At the time, I still weighed only 100 pounds, but my eating habits had gotten better. The doctors stressed that it was important for me to have family meals, but during a family therapy session, my mother confessed that she did not feel like she could handle the pressure because she worked until eight at night. So I moved into my dad's home. For a while, I was doing okay, but then eating became stressful again—there were just too many choices—and I started backsliding and eating less. It wasn't long before my weight was back down to 88 pounds.

During the summer before my junior year, I was seeing a new doctor who warned me that unless I turned things around, I would have to go back to the hospital. I knew I needed to gain weight if I was going to make it to college, but after all those years of unhealthy eating, I didn't know how. That's when I started bingeing. Eating during the day was too stressful, so I'd fast all day, then eat 2,000 to 7,000 calories' worth of food at night—mostly cookies, waffles, cereal, and peanut butter—and go to sleep so I wouldn't have to think about it. Then I'd wake up and start all over again. Naturally, I started gaining weight—I put on about 40 pounds during the school year. Every two weeks or so, I'd see my mom, and she'd tell me I looked nice. Everyone around me was so excited that I was no longer stick-thin, but the bingeing made me feel out of control and horrible about myself. I managed to graduate from high school and go off to college, but I was stuck in a vicious cycle and couldn't stop.

Breaking the Cycle

So after two years of bingeing, I became anorexic again. Bouncing between the two extremes became my pattern. I had to be hospitalized two more times, most recently in Arizona in the spring of 2001. The doctors and therapists there were able to make me see how I had to change my way of thinking about food, and I finally reached a turning point. Since then, my treatment has been going well—I'm in therapy, and I also take medication for anxiety and depression. I still eat most of my calories at night—although I will drink a smoothie for lunch—but I'm working on overcoming that habit.

At the age of 20, my eating is very different than it ever has been: I no longer consider any food bad or completely off-limits. My weight has stabilized at 115, and I feel okay about that, even though my mom always told me that she weighed 110 in college and we're the same height. Recovering from an entrenched eating disorder can take a long time, but I'm at a point where I'm trying to stop judging my bad eating habits and start figuring out what else is troubling me.

At the moment, I don't have much of a relationship with my mother. I speak to her maybe once a month and see her even less frequently. For years, I tried to get her to look at some of her own issues with food, but she has resisted. I love her very much, and I think she's a wonderful person in many ways, but because she hasn't been a healthy influence, I feel that I need to keep my distance for now. My father and step-mother have been supportive, and someday, I hope my mother and I will be closer in a healthy way. In the meantime, I'm trying to find ways to nurture myself. I live with a friend in New York City and work full-time as a sales rep for a marketing company, plus I'm going to college part-time, so my life is really busy. I feel confident that I will be able to overcome my eating disorders. It'll just take some time.

I Survived Breast Cancer

Julianne Buescher

According to the National Cancer Institute, approximately 13 percent of all women will be diagnosed with breast cancer at some point in their lives. Although diagnostic techniques and treatments have improved significantly since the 1970s, cancer rates have gone up steadily because Americans are living longer than ever before. For some women the threat of breast cancer is even higher because of family history. For these women, getting the disease seems inevitable. In the following selection Julianne Buescher describes her battle with the disease that almost took her life and the lives of her mother and grandmother. With wit and humor, she describes her own long fight to survive surgery and chemotherapy and the strategies that she used to cope with the loss of her breasts, ovaries, and hair. In the end, even after a recurrence of the disease, which spread to her lymph nodes, she refers to herself as a survivor and a warrior. Buescher is an independent filmmaker, whose recent project Resculpting Venus *is a comic look at her trials with breast cancer.*

"Where do you think you're going?" screeched the cancer-walk volunteer, planting himself in front of the opening to the giant pink tent. He tugged at his hot pink T-shirt, which was covered with a collection of buttons he must have picked up at every Southern California cancer event for the past ten years.

"Oh," I squeaked, trying not to giggle. "Actually, I really need some water." It was only 9 a.m., but already incredibly hot outside, and the walk was about to start. I moved to go inside to reach the haven packed with shade, snacks, tables full of freebies, and yes—water.

Julianne Buescher, New Venus.com, "The Breast Defense Is a Good Offense," *Bust*, Spring 2002, pp. 56, 58–61. Copyright © 1999 by Julianne Buescher. Original title "Survive This." Reproduced by permission of the author.

He thrust his hands on his hips and said slowly, so that I was sure to understand, "THIS tent is ONLY for SURVIVORS!"

I totally clenched. I could feel my eyes pressing into glaring slits and the corners of my mouth curling up. As I stretched my fingers, my knuckles cracked and I, too, put my fists to my hips. Only for survivors, huh? I gave a little "look who's messing with the wrong grrrl" huff as we tried to stare each other down, and then I did the unthinkable, as usual.

Okay, okay—how was this poor sap supposed to know that I'd had my breasts and ovaries removed five years ago? I suppose I could have let him off easy and just hung my head low and played the pity card. I mean, all he saw in front of him was this spunky girl all Urban-Outfitted out who's obviously trying to sneak in and grab a bag full of free s**t not meant for someone who looks like me, right? But just what does a "survivor" look like, anyway?. . .

Hand-Me-Down Genes

Cancer—and spunk—run in my family. Twenty-four years ago, my Mom had her breasts removed and my Grandma, who just turned 88, had breast cancer, too, over forty years ago. So it's always been a part of my life, in one way or another, but never in a silent, scary way. I remember being very little when Grandma took us swimming. I could see her scars behind the flopping empty cups of her bathing suit. She would plainly and honestly tell her story, devoid of shame and pity and fear. I thought she was the most beautiful, powerful warrior in the world.

We would talk about Mom's surgery, too, and eventually came the point when I realized my turn was coming up fast.

I started getting annual mammograms in my early twenties. I picked a doctor who understood my family history, and didn't tell me I was "too young to worry about it." We got along great! And he was so cool about my practical jokes.

Well, until that one visit, when I put a remote control fart machine under his chair.

"Umm. . .Julianne, I. . ."

phhhhhhhphphtt

". . .I looked over your x-rays and. . ."

pllpphheerrt

". . .and the results from your biopsy. . ."

puurrrrfffff

"I need to tell you that. . ."

poit

"Julianne! The biopsy came back positive! You have cancer."

We sat for a moment. I think he expected me to cry. I triggered off one last mechanical fart. Then, I took a small cassette player from my bag and placed it on his desk. He let loose all the techno-garble about my new condition into the recorder. We even managed a few chuckles here and there. There were no tissues left when we were done—he had used them all. . . .

Researching Options

I called Grandma and told her I got it. Cancer—in the right breast. "Oh, that's where I got mine!" she recalled. "And then, five years later, why, I got it in the other breast! Yup. And the same thing happened to your mother." She also told me how the hospitals didn't have any sort of prosthetics back then. "Well, I had to make my own fake boobie. I filled a sock with bird seed, and it made a great match."

I suddenly saw myself sitting in front of the boob tube in a powder-blue housecoat, and cat-eye glasses. I was scolding my parakeet for pecking at my seed-filled tittie-sock as I tried to watch the latest "I Love Lucy" episode.

That's when I decided to have both of my breasts removed at the same time.

I dove into bookstores, libraries, hospitals, the Web; I read, watched, and listened to everything I could get my hands on. Soon I knew exactly what I wanted to do. It was time to shop for a surgeon.

The first one I called sounded shocked when I explained that I wanted a bilateral mastectomy. "Oh I get it," he said, re-assuring himself, "you're calling for your bubba, right honey?"

"No," I replied, "for me."

"What? You sound so young!" I sighed, "Yeah, I'm 28."

"Twenty-eight?" he yelped, "there goes *your* social life!" I hung up the phone and dialed the next number. . . .

Facing a Double Mastectomy

Sitting down with yourself to face the possibility of your own death can, basically, suck. It was so easy for me to lay across that pile of books on the floor and just not care about any of it anymore. Dark little ideas with pointy tails started to pop up on my "things I could actually do if I really wanted to" list. Things like "go into a really deep depression" or "try a swift and easy suicide." I lay sprawled across my books, considering the options. . . .

That next morning, in a matter of hours, I'd have my eight-year-old figure back. I'd be able to do yoga, archery, even jog; everything my D-cuppers had kept me from enjoying for so long. Of course, that wasn't something to share with my Dad as he paced back and forth next to my pre-op gurney. What could I say, except, "I'm glad you're here!" (He'd flown in from Ohio that morning). "Mom wanted to be here, too," he stumbled. "But she's afraid of flying," I finished. "Well, at least we're together for Thanksgiving!" I added. Dad stopped pacing. "I have to leave. Grandpa died yesterday; I have to get back for the funeral." Who? And my what? And you're huh?

That's when he asked me to come home to recover. My eyes went wide—all I could see was me in a hideous yellow gown in the middle of a field, flanked by giggling teens. A guy in a bright blue tux announces that I'm runner up for Corn Queen, and the winning teen is promptly crowned with a cob-shaped tiara.

I stared at my Dad and shook my head. A smiling nurse swept in carrying IV bags. "Hey, are those my new boobs?" I quipped. My Dad started to cry.

When I awoke, the nurse was waggling a gobbling turkey doll in my face. "This is for you! We all think you're so brave!" she cooed. I tried to lift my arm to wave the turkey out of my face. Ouch! Nurse Liddy kept on talking. "The first night alone is the worst, but I'll be at your house to take care of you, okay? We'll have such fun!" Dad looked grateful, as he slurped down the rest of my Jello. I just sort of nodded and went back to sleep. . . .

The Cancer Had Spread

The holidays that year were full of new shopping adventures. I had decided not to get reconstruction (even *more* surgery? No thanks!), so I was out and about looking for a new pair of falsies. I mean, out here in Hollywood everyone's are fake, anyway—so what's the diff? The diff, I soon discovered, was that I had become a "specialty case." I would have to go to "specialty" stores, and get "specialty" catalogues in the mail, that arrived sealed discreetly in big pink envelopes. . . .

F**k! Just when I thought I was home free, I found out that the cancer had spread to my lymph nodes. "Not many; only two out of 13 nodes are involved," my surgeon explained, "and only a few cells in each." I had already decided to remove my ovaries; that would stop the hormones from triggering any future cancer growth. Mom and Grandma did that, too, and I knew that's why they were still around. But for me, it wouldn't be enough. I'd need the big guns. Chemotherapy. The word bounced around in my skull. I decided I could handle it.

I looked up at my surgeon to tell him, suddenly noticing his slick, bald head. That's when I screamed.

Three Months of Chemotherapy

I had become officially, absolutely "special." And I suddenly longed to talk with other women who were going through the same thing I was. I started visiting a handful of support groups around town, and, although I did get lots of great info and met lots of people, I never did find a place to fit in. I'd listen to the women, all over 50, talk about their husbands, the cruises they were planning, how cute their grandchildren were. They would just sort of wince when I told them I wanted to tattoo my scars. I couldn't talk to them about dating, or my career, or what to do when your boob falls out while swing dancing. I couldn't possibly be *this* unique, could I? I felt like I was traveling into a whole new life, and nobody had a map. There were no young women, no young women's groups, no books about young women—I was on this island alone. I'd have to make the whole thing up as I went along. I was angry, I was frustrated, and, for the first time in my life, I was scared. Really, really scared. And the worst thing was, I had to admit to myself that I needed somebody. I needed my Mom. And nothing could scare a grown woman more.

In a matter of weeks, I had lost all—I mean *all*—of my hair. I stood in front of the mirror, bald and breastless. I didn't choose to get sick, but I chose everything about getting well. Every moment. Would I get up today? Yes. Would I keep my breakfast down? Yes. Would I audition for Star Trek? Yes! But as I ran my fingers across the scars on my chest, and lightly rubbed my scalp, I wondered if there would ever be anyone who could really understand what I was going through, anyone who could really even care.

"Honey, is my bathrobe in here?" It was Mom! She'd already been staying with me a month (she took the train), but she hadn't yet seen my scars. I awkwardly turned to face her. Without a word, she unbuttoned her top. I'd never seen her scars, either. We looked at each other, smiling weakly. I reached out to touch the thin layer of skin that barely covered her ribs, and I saw her heart move. We fell into each others arms and stayed there, silently swaying, tears dripping along each other's chests.

Am I the daughter of warriors? Yes! . . .

I had so much fun those three months of chemo. Mom and I would play Scrabble while I got the four-hour drip. We would experiment in the kitchen, creating new "cancer chick" recipes. We'd go together to my auditions and recording jobs. We giggled for hours when I won awards for my breast-packed role in that musical. And I even won a "Paint-Yourself-DayGlo" contest by turning my bald head into a black-lit skull with an eight ball in the center. I felt great. I actually bought pens that were shaped like chemo syringes, and used them to write my first film: a comedy about breast cancer. Something wonderful had happened. Something clicked. I was blossoming, from somewhere deeper than I'd ever felt. And when the chemo was over, and Mom went back home, I knew it was safe to keep blooming. I felt so truly alive.

I'm a Survivor

My "Things To Do Tomorrow" list became a "What's Today's Adventure?" challenge. Snowboarding, skydiving, Japanese sword fighting, ukulele playing, or smaller things, like visiting a new café for lunch, or taking a different road home. I wondered what I could do differently every day to expand and change my world, even if it meant shaking up someone else's. Even if it meant doing the unthinkable. . . .

I guess I'll always be the different one, making it up as I go. It's really all any of us can do. And whatever we might call each other—survivor, warrior, kicker-of-various-asses—I can't imagine anything more unthinkable than not being ourselves. That's something worth fighting for. So, it looks like I'm on this island until I decide I'm ready to leave. Stirring it up, and playing hard. After all, isn't that what "special" girls do?

My Journey Through Postpartum Depression

Brooke Shields

Only recently has postpartum depression (PPD), a severe mood disorder that some women develop after giving birth, been considered a serious medical condition. Approximately half a million women suffer from PPD each year. For years PPD was referred to as the "baby blues" and considered a normal part of the childbirth cycle. It is now recognized as a devastating mental illness that can lead to irrational behavior, even suicide and infanticide. Following a terrifying ordeal with PPD, well-known actress Brooke Shields wrote a book chronicling her journey. In Down Came the Rain, *Shields describes the lengths she took to conceive her daughter and the nightmarish months that followed when she felt she could not bond with her baby and felt overwhelmed, scared, and depressed. In the following excerpt she describes the first several weeks after the delivery during which she cried nearly all day long and could barely perform the necessary duties to care for her newborn. She could not talk about her emotional pain with anyone, not even her husband Chris.*

As I walked barefoot into our apartment, carrying my newborn, I felt disoriented. When I had left this space five days ago, I was a totally different person. Now, passing through the same doors, I had become a mother, and the world, as I related to it, had entirely changed. As I held my five-day-old baby girl in my arms, I looked around the apartment and thought, Where am I? It was like being in the Twilight Zone, and I kept waiting for someone to turn off the TV.

Chris and I were suddenly alone with a brand-new baby, and we weren't sure what to do. We stared at each other for a while and then tried to settle in. I changed into a pair of Chris's shorts, which were the only thing that fit over the girdle I had to wear as a result of the C-section. My legs were far from shorts-worthy, but I tried not to think about that. I was just happy to be out of my dress. We put the little one in a Moses basket. Then, in an attempt to gain control, I decided to unpack immediately and tidy up the house. Chris kindly reminded me that I'd just had a baby and the tidying up could wait. He ordered me to bed and added that once we all got some sleep, I could neaten to my heart's desire. He was under the impression that the baby would drift off into a peaceful slumber and we would all get caught up on the sleep we had been deprived of in the hospital. I must admit that I, too, naively believed that because we were home and away from constant interruptions, rest was imminent. Almost every mother I knew had let her new baby sleep at least one night in the hospital nursery before going home so the mom could launch into baby land slightly rested. Since we were too afraid of the press or even of a staff member sneaking photos of Rowan, we never let her out of our sight. Consequently, neither Chris nor I had really slept in five days, and we were feeling quite beaten up because of it. Unfortunately we soon found out that being home hardly provided the respite we craved. . . .

Panic, Fear, and Devastation

At first I thought what I was feeling was just exhaustion, but with it came an overriding sense of panic that I had never felt before. Rowan kept crying, and I began to dread the moment when Chris would bring her back to me. I started to experience a sick sensation in my stomach; it was as if a vise were tightening around my chest. Instead of the nervous anxiety that often accompanies panic, a feeling of devastation overcame me. I hardly moved. Sitting on my bed, I let out a deep, slow, guttural wail. I wasn't simply emotional or weepy, like I had been told I might be. This was something quite different. In the past, if I got depressed or if I felt sad or down, I knew I could counteract it with exercise, a good night's sleep, or a nice dinner with a friend. If PMS made me introspective or melancholy, or if the pressures of life made me gloomy, I knew these feelings wouldn't last forever. But this was sadness of a shockingly different magnitude. It felt as if it would never go away.

In general, I have always loved babies, and Rowan was not only amazing and alert but also quite beautiful. Her features were perfectly formed, and she looked like an angel. But I felt no appreciation for the little miracle. Although I didn't dislike her, I wasn't sure I wanted her living with us. In addition, I could hardly stand on my own two feet because of the sheer mass and weight of my body. . . .

I tried to rationalize that I was physically impaired and should give myself a break, but I didn't have any desire to power through and care for this baby. I got hit with a wave of self-defeat and self-loathing and had an urge to smash my head against the wall repeatedly. Chris told me to get off my feet and back into bed. Once there, my crying recommenced, and I started strongly believing that I couldn't be a mother. I was already proving to be incompetent, and we hadn't been home a day! What had I done? Why didn't I want to be near my baby?

I had little time to contemplate such thoughts, because it was time for Rowan to eat again (or snack, I should say). Without the help of a nurse or a lactation specialist, I was in trouble once more. I accepted Chris's help as he guided the baby's mouth onto my nipple; this time I didn't become annoyed or impatient with him or myself. I sat there almost catatonically, staring out into space. Rowan's nursing made me feel drugged and temporarily comforted me. But the moment she was finished and taken from me, I started to sob once more. I sat up with my huge legs stretched out in front of me and, slowly rocking back and forth with my face up toward the ceiling, my arms limp at my sides, I sobbed. I couldn't stop. What was I going to do? Was I ever going to stop feeling like this? Misery enveloped me. . . .

After only a couple of days of being home, my crying had increased and no longer occurred only in between feedings but during them as well. At times I even had trouble holding Rowan because of my choking sobs. Why was I crying more than my baby? Here I was, finally the mother of a beautiful baby girl I had worked so hard to have, and I felt like my life was over. Where was the bliss? Where was the happiness that I had expected to feel by becoming a mother? She was my baby; the baby I had wanted for so long. Why didn't I feel remotely comforted by having or holding her? I had always felt that a baby was the one major thing missing from my life, that a child would complete the picture and bring everything into focus. Once I was a mother, the different parts of my world would all converge, and I would experience life as I'd envisioned it and in turn would know what I was meant to be. But having a baby clouded my vision and threatened whatever peace had already existed. Instead of wanting to move forward, all I wanted was for life to return to the way it was before I had Rowan. . . .

Unable to Bond

I felt no connection to my daughter and wanted to die because of it. She grew inside my body, for God's sake, and I didn't even feel related to her. I had always thought I would immediately feel closer to my child than I did to anybody else in my life. I'd thought we would be undeniably bonded from the moment I laid eyes on her. What was wrong with me? What a horrible mother I was! Her cry didn't annoy me or grate on my nerves, but it also didn't register with me, either. I felt numb to it. I practically had to strain to hear her voice, which seemed so far away, even though she was in the adjoining room and the door was open. I could almost justify not hearing it.

My profound detachment made me suffer unbearably, and I believed I had nowhere to turn. I remember looking out of the bedroom window and envisioning myself jumping. I concluded that it wouldn't be too effective, because we weren't high enough. This upset me even more. The frightening part was that my thoughts were extremely rational. They made clear sense to me. It felt like an appealing option to erase myself from this life. What would stop me from acting on any of these thoughts? I needed and wanted a way out. My mind was full of visions of escape, and these constantly overshadowed thoughts about my miraculous baby girl.

During what was becoming one of the darkest points in my life, I sat holding my newborn and could not avoid the image of her flying through the air and hitting the wall in front of me. I had no desire to hurt my baby and didn't see myself as the one throwing her, thank God, but the wall morphed into a video game, and in it her little body smacked the surface and slid down onto the floor. I was horrified, and although I knew deep in my soul that I would not harm her, the image all but destroyed me.

I was desperate to have a natural and healthy connection with my daughter, but it was feeling so forced. It was as if I were trapped behind a thick glass wall. I had never felt apathy in my life, and when I had least expected it, it crept in and took over. I couldn't shake the feeling of doom and gloom that pervaded each moment. I was afraid of myself and felt threatened by the dangerous thoughts running so calmly through my head. They all felt too real. When would I wake up from this bad dream? . . .

Seeking Help

When it was time to take myself and the baby for our first postpartum visit, Rowan was as quiet as a mouse, while I was

the one who broke down. It quickly turned into a lengthy
mommy checkup. While the baby sat with Chris and a nurse,
Dr. Rebarber guided me into an empty exam room so we
could talk. I told him I was not doing well at all and explained through my sobs that I couldn't take care of this baby.
I just didn't want to do it. I told him that I felt I had no relationship to her. Because I felt so ashamed, I probably sounded
stronger than I felt. He said to trust him, that this feeling
would pass and that many new mothers went through the
baby blues. He explained that it had to do with the fact that
out with the placenta went many of the hormones contributing to the sense of well-being I had felt during the pregnancy.
Once the hormones equalized, I would start feeling better. He
said the hormonal shifts that occur postpartum are often a
shock to women, but even his wife went through it, and it was
very normal. He, too, suggested that I not breast-feed. I
couldn't even explain my theory on why I needed to keep doing it. He was so warm and caring, and he had been right
about everything before. I stopped crying long enough to admit that I felt I had made a mistake by having a baby. He
looked at me seriously and said, "You know what, Brooke? I'm
not God. I can only do my best, but if that baby was not
meant to be here, she wouldn't be." He had sure seemed god-
like to me when he so adeptly saved my daughter's life, as well
as my own, so I decided to trust him, once again. Maybe it
was hormonal, or maybe I was one of those emotional women
who was making more out of it than necessary. Even though
it appeared to be more serious than a hormonal imbalance, I
would try mind over matter. I felt too ashamed to keep trying
to convince him it was otherwise. The doctor said he would
keep checking on me and that it might help if I talked to
other mothers I knew and got their perspective. In addition to
referring us to a pediatrician, he suggested we both come back
in a week. Rowan would surely be fine, but to me a week

sounded like an eternity. We left the office and I tried to feel encouraged.

As I reentered the apartment, the same feelings came flooding in like a bursting of Hoover Dam. My friend Sherie came over with a stack of information on postpartum depression that she'd printed out from the Internet. She explained that everything I had said to her on the phone was repeated practically verbatim in this material. She also brought me two books on different women's accounts—one from the early 1990s and one that looked like a medical textbook—and begged me to page through them. I couldn't imagine that any of the material could possibly have anything to do with me. Plus, the last thing I wanted to do was read information about other people's lives or on how "common" my feelings were. I was certain that nobody else could possibly feel what I was feeling. She might as well have been giving me information on penile enlargement; it was that irrelevant to me. Postpartum depression was a crazy person's affliction, and I associated it only with those people who harmed their kids by doing things like driving the car into a lake. I was certainly not in that category. I had no intention of ever harming my baby, although I also didn't seem to have any intention of becoming attached to her, either. I was a healthy-minded and capable woman who simply shouldn't have had a child. Postpartum depression was plainly not something that affected someone like me. It hit only those people you read about in the news. . . .

Since my checkup, Dr. Rebarber had been phoning me daily to see how I was doing. During one of his calls, he told me that while almost all women experienced some form of the baby blues, many also suffered from the more acute postpartum depression. He had been thinking about the look on my face and about what I'd said to him regarding my mood, and because it sounded so severe and so out of character, he suggested I might want to see a therapist and even try some medication. . . . I had been considering a therapist but hadn't followed through. As far as medication was concerned, it was out of the question, because I was still breastfeeding and had no intention of stopping. Dr. Rebarber explained that there was medicine I could take that wouldn't get into my milk or affect the baby. I said I had to think about it but did not like the idea of taking medicine. None of the women I knew of had needed medication after giving birth, and I felt I shouldn't, either. In my entire life, I had never needed drugs to help with my moods and didn't want to start now. It was yet another sign of my weakness and failure as a mother. I hung up the phone feeling even more hopeless, like I was being tortured. This was indeed a losing battle.

I told my husband about Dr. Rebarber's suggestions, and he exhaled with relief. Maybe more help did exist. Chris knew I was upset at the prospect of taking drugs, so he gently explained that many people took medication for a myriad of reasons and that there was nothing wrong with it. It wouldn't have to be forever, and if it made me feel better, it was worth a try. In under three weeks, I had managed to terrify everyone who cared for me, and now my husband wanted me to become a pill popper!. . . I couldn't face the thought of being dependent on medication to feel better, especially when all my dreams had supposedly just come true by having a baby.

How I Made Peace With My Secondary Infertility

Julie Stiegemeyer

Secondary infertility, or the inability to conceive or maintain a second pregnancy after the successful birth of a child, is thought to be more common than primary fertility. There can be a number of reasons for secondary infertility, such as endometriosis, prior or current pelvic or fallopian tube infections, or maternal age. Women who suffer from this condition are not always taken seriously by health care providers or by other women who feel that because the sufferers already have a child, their current condition is not a serious issue. In the following selection Julie Stiegemeyer writes about her struggle to come to terms with not being able to give birth to a second child. At first she did not understand the condition, but after months of research she finally learned that she had endometriosis most likely caused by incomplete healing after her cesarean section and a lump on her thyroid gland. Following corrective surgeries, she and her husband hoped for the best. Unfortunately, over six years later, she and her husband have not yet conceived a second child. However, Stiegemeyer has come to terms with not being able to add to her small family, and she attributes her great strength in battling this emotional and physical rollercoaster to her husband and her faith in God. Stiegemeyer is a poet and the author of several children's books.

Our first son was born in 1995, an "accident" who turned out to be our "miracle baby." You hear about couples who try for years to conceive and finally—after months and months and months—have the child of their dreams, their miracle baby. Our miracle baby came before my husband and I knew we had a problem.

About two and a half years after he was born, we were ready for child number two to make our family "complete"— one son, one daughter, a mom, a dad—the perfect package. However, after a few months, I began to get worried. Why was this taking so long?

My gynecologist immediately put me on fertility drugs, which made me edgy. With a toddler at home and a husband often traveling for work, I found dealing with these side effects increasingly difficult. After some months went by, I decided to see an infertility specialist. He was a wonderfully reassuring grandfather type who helped me to remember that yes, we had one child; conceiving the second had a good chance of happening, too.

One day soon, I thought, I'd finally have that positive pregnancy test. Before much longer, I'd be able to call our family and friends to tell them our son was going to be a big brother. But the pregnancy tests were always negative; our second child was never conceived.

Secondary Infertility Defined

Those unable to conceive a child after 12 months without contraception are considered to have primary infertility, as defined by the Centers for Disease Control [CDC]. According to a 1995 survey by the CDC, 6.1 million American women ages 15 through 44 experience impaired ability to have children.

Surprisingly, the CDC report on infertility revealed that more than half the women of reproductive age who experience infertility already have at least one child. These couples experience secondary infertility, which refers to the inability to have another child after at least 12 months of trying. Resolve, Inc., the national infertility association, estimates more than three million Americans struggle with secondary infertility.

"Even though secondary infertility is more prevalent than primary infertility, couples are less apt to seek treatment for this condition," reports Resolve, Inc. "When their first child is conceived with ease, many couples are caught completely off guard by the difficulty of having a second child, because they believe past fertility insures future fertility."

Caught off guard is definitely the way I'd describe how my husband and I felt when we realized just how difficult it would be to have our dreamed-for second child. The infertility specialist I saw performed tests that showed extensive endometriosis [growth of uterine lining outside the uterus,] (probably caused by incomplete healing after my C-section) and found a nodule on my thyroid gland. We coordinated the two surgeries—the thyroid surgery and a laparoscopy to "clean out" the endometriosis—and my mom came to help take care of our son.

Post-surgery, our hopes soared. Surely now we'd have no problem conceiving. But the months wore on, the doctor visits were frequent (and difficult to manage with a toddler), and the medical expenses added up. We found our insurance coverage was less extensive than we were led to believe.

Soon thereafter, my husband and I had "the talk," one step in coming to terms with our infertility. We talked about the emotional toll the treatments caused, the strain on our marriage, and the frustration of not enjoying our son's childhood because we were so wrapped up in having another child. We decided to take a break from treatment.

My physician said, "If you stop treatment, your chances of pregnancy are extremely low." My husband said, "Our family is in God's hands. Let's trust him to know the best size for our family." My heart said, *Lord, I can't handle this treatment roller coaster anymore. It's in your hands.*

Understanding the Condition

When we first couldn't conceive, I turned to my gynecologist, then to a reproductive endocrinologist to help me understand my infertility and improve our chances for another child. Then I researched and educated myself about all the fancy doctor-speak: polycystic ovarian syndrome, fibroids, Clomid, etc. A simple Google search led to many resources on understanding primary and secondary infertility. Resolve, Inc. provided extremely helpful information. Understanding what to expect from my testing and treatment helped prepare me emotionally to deal with what was to come.

Frequently those who experience secondary infertility feel caught "in the middle." It's hard to talk to friends who have no children and are experiencing infertility because they think, *You already have a child. Be grateful for him.* It's also difficult to talk to moms who have two or more kids because they think, *What I wouldn't give for the free time and quiet of a one-child household!* This can make a couple feel more isolated in their struggle; that's why it's so important to find support through organizations such as Resolve, Inc.

Many couples who deal with secondary infertility feel sad as their only child grows older. It's bittersweet to watch our son go through the stages of childhood and know we'll experience these only once. Milestones like his first loose tooth, his first day of kindergarten, or the day he learned to ride his bike came and went so quickly. While I love watching him grow and gain independence, I also feel sad that I'll never experience these special days with another child. In a sense, our empty nest came too quickly.

Related to this concern for many is the issue of child spacing. As the child in the family grows older, the couple must decide how many years to prolong fertility treatments, resulting in a wider gap between children. The age of the couple affects childbearing, but another factor involved with secondary infertility is how far apart to space children.

For the couple experiencing secondary infertility, they must deal with disappointment and loss; however, their child must cope with the issues as well. Couples may struggle with "letting down" each other, but have the additional burden of feeling as though they've denied their child the blessing of having a sibling.

"It's quite possible that children pick up on the societal norm for families and realize that their family is somehow different. It's painful to feel that your child is being set apart or deprived," says Harriet Fishman Simons, author of *Wanting Another Child: Coping with Secondary Infertility.* "Mom—why can't I have a baby brother or sister?" becomes the refrain for many only children. Explaining to a child that families come in all sizes and pointing out the positives of their only-child status can alleviate some of the frustrations and fears of the couple as well as of their child.

I'd always assumed that if I had any children, I'd have more than one. I grew up with two brothers, and while my husband and I never imagined having a large family, we hoped for at least two kids. Struggling with this "definition" of family is something with which many people experiencing secondary infertility must grapple. As Simons writes, "While on some level couples know they and a single child are a family, it may not always feel like what a 'real family' should be. As the adoptive mother of a second child put it, yes, one child does make a family, but 'two is more of a family.'"

In one sense, my emotional struggle with secondary infertility was more about recreating my expectations of an ideal family; that four-person ideal was going to have to go. As Simons notes, "You may need to grieve for the fantasized family you may be unable to have before you're able to refocus on choosing alternative outcomes."

Finding Resolution

Couples who experience secondary infertility come through their experience in at least three ways. Some couples, after seeking treatment, ultimately have the second child they hoped for. Others may build their family through adoption. Still others come to the conclusion that having an only child (or fewer children) is enough.

It takes time to sort through the muddle of emotions associated with secondary infertility. It's been almost six years since we first sought treatment. While my husband and I would still love a second child, we have found contentment in our family of three and no longer want to go through the stress and difficulties of treatment. The twinges of sorrow are still with me, but mostly, they're only twinges. After holding a friend's new baby or after hearing a stray comment ("Is he your only child?"), I still can be shaken from my normal composure.

But good things have come from our only-child status. Life is simpler with only one sports and music lesson schedule to juggle. Our son may never wear the "I'm the big brother" T-shirt, but we also don't have to deal with sibling rivalry and bickering. Taking care of cooking and laundry are easier. While it made me sad to send my son off to school because I had no little one at home, I relish the free time I have during the day now. That extra time has given me the opportunity to do volunteer work with the PTA and at church, and to pursue my lifelong love of writing.

Remember Hannah, the Old Testament mother of the prophet Samuel? She prayed: "O Lord Almighty, if you will only look upon your servant's misery and remember me, and not forget your servant but give her a son, then I will give him to the Lord for all the days of his life" (1 Samuel 1:11). Hannah, Abraham's wife, Sarah, and other women in the Bible also struggled with infertility. I've prayed the same prayers they did. I've had the same longing as theirs. Knowing I'm not alone in my struggle—that other women felt the same grief and sorrow over infertility—helps me cope.

Most important, though, I'm forced to cling to my Savior. At times I've felt anger and frustration toward God for not answering our prayers the way I think they should be answered. But now, years later, I honestly can say struggling through secondary infertility has been a blessing.

Instead of resenting what we haven't been given, I've learned to become more grateful to God for the blessings we do have, including our marriage, our precious son, and, most important, salvation in Christ. I know now that God can bring good out of difficulties. I've learned, in a small way, that contentment is not something I can create within myself. Contentment is a gift of God, and I cling to him for all good gifts. Mostly, I'm reassured that God truly has sustained our family and continues to do so. He cares for me through all the changes and situations in my life. Psalm 55:22 has proven true for me: "Cast your cares on the Lord and he will sustain you." What more can I hope for?

Organizations to Contact

American Fertility Association (AFA)
666 Fifth Ave., Suite 278, New York, NY 10103
(888) 917-3777 • fax: (718) 601-7722
e-mail: info@theafa.org
Web site: www.theafa.org

The AFA is a national nonprofit organization that provides support for women facing fertility problems. It offers online chat boards, support and referral services, and information to educate the public about reproductive diseases. The AFA publishes *infocus*, a quarterly magazine that focuses on specific fertility issues.

American Medical Women's Association (AMWA)
801 North Fairfax St., Suite 400, Alexandria, VA 22314
(703) 838-0500 • fax: (703) 549-3864
Web site: www.amwa-doc.org

Founded in 1915, the AMWA is composed of over ten thousand female doctors and medical students. The AMWA works on the local, national, and international level to educate the public about women's health issues and to advance women in medicine by providing and developing leadership, advocacy, and education. The AMWA regularly publishes two periodicals, the *Journal of the American Medical Women's Association* and *AMWA Connections.*

American Society for Reproductive Medicine (ASRM)
1209 Montgomery Hwy., Birmingham, AL 35216
(205) 978-5000 • fax: (205) 978-5005
e-mail: asrm@asrm.org
Web site: www.asrm.org

The ASRM is a nonprofit organization that brings together health care providers who specialize in reproductive medicine. In addition to acting as a collective voice for its members, the

ASRM also serves as an advocate and educator for the lay public. The ASRM regularly publishes its newsletter *ASRM Bulletins* and reports on current issues in fertility treatments.

International Women's Health Coalition (IWHC)

333 Seventh Ave., Sixth Fl., New York, NY 10001
(212) 979-8500 • fax: (212) 979-9009
e-mail: info@iwhc.org
Web site: www.iwhc.org

Founded in 1984, the IWHC works toward educating the world about women's reproductive rights and sexual health issues. The IWHC provides financial support for various organizations around the world, helps provide women with access to contraception and safe abortions, and advocates for the reproductive freedom of girls and women. Recent publications include *Unfair and Unbalanced: Women, Health, and U.S. Foreign Policy* and *Positively Informed: Lesson Plans and Guidance for Sexuality Educators and Advocates.*

National Association of Anorexia Nervosa and Associated Disorders (ANAD)

PO Box 7, Highland, IL 60035
(847) 831-3438
e-mail: anad20@aol.com
Web site: www.anad.org

Founded in 1976, the ANAD offers free hotline counseling, a national network of support groups, referrals to health care professionals, and education and prevention programs concerning eating disorders. In addition, the ANAD undertakes and encourages research, fights advertising that encourages unhealthy body images, and organizes advocacy campaigns to protect potential victims of eating disorders.

National Women's Health Information Center (NWHIC)

8550 Arlington Blvd., Suite 300, Fairfax, VA 22031
(800) 994-WOMAN
Web site: www.4woman.gov

Sponsored by the Office of Women's Health and the U.S. Department of Health and Human Services, the NWHIC offers information through their Web site and call center on over eight hundred women's health topics. The main goals of NWHIC include educating health professionals and motivating consumers to change poor health-related behaviors. In addition to pamphlets and reports, the NWHIC publishes the monthly newsletter *Healthy Women Today*.

National Women's Health Network (NWHN)
514 10th St. NW, Suite 400, Washington, DC   20004
(202) 347-1140 • fax: (202) 347-1168
e-mail: nwhn@nwhn.org
Web site: www.womenshealthnetwork.org

Since 1975 the NWHN has worked toward promoting health and wellness for women. The NWHN focuses on women's reproductive and sexual health, changing cultural perceptions of menopause, and working toward establishing a universal health care system to meet the needs of women. In addition to the bimonthly newsletter *Women's Health Activist*, the NWHN publishes a number of reports and documents relating to women's health.

National Women's Health Resource Center (NWHRC)
120 Albany St., Suite 820, New Brunswick, NJ   08901
(877) 986-9472
Web site: www.healthywomen.org

The NWHRC is a nonprofit organization dedicated to helping women make informed decisions about their health. As a national clearinghouse for women's health information, the NWHRC attempts to provide information that is comprehensive and objective. The NWHRC's publications cover many aspects of women's health and most of them are available for free on the organization's Web site.

Resolve: The National Infertility Association
1310 Broadway, Somerville, MA   02144
(888) 623-0744
e-mail: info@resolve.org
Web site: www.resolve.org

Established in 1974, Resolve is a nonprofit organization that seeks to educate the public about reproductive issues. In addition, Resolve offers support for women suffering from reproductive disorders with the goal of helping all potential parents achieve their goals. Resolve has published a variety of reports about infertility, including *Miscarriage: The Hidden Loss.*

Susan G. Komen Breast Cancer Foundation
5005 LBJ Fwy., Suite 520, Dallas, TX   75244
(800) 462-9273 • fax: (972) 855-1605
Web site: www.komen.org

The Susan G. Komen Breast Cancer Foundation was founded in 1982 by Nancy Goodman Brinker after her sister Susan died from breast cancer. Since then it has become one of the leading organizations in the fight against breast cancer by sponsoring educational seminars, fund-raising events, and breast cancer research. In addition to a variety of reports on current breast cancer issues, the foundation also provides a support forum for women with breast cancer.

Bibliography

Books

Linda Lewis Alexander et al.	*New Dimensions in Women's Health.* 3rd ed. Sudbury, MA: Jones and Bartlett, 2004.
Christine Ammer	*The Encyclopedia of Women's Health.* 5th ed. New York: Facts On File, 2005.
Boston Women's Health Book Collective	*Our Bodies, Ourselves: A New Edition for a New Era.* 35th anniversary ed. New York: Simon & Schuster. 2005.
Gwyneth Boswell and Fiona Poland, eds.	*Women's Minds, Women's Bodies: Interdisciplinary Approaches to Women's Health.* New York: Palgrave Macmillan, 2003.
Karen J. Carlson, Stephanie A. Eisenstat, and Terra Ziporyn	*The New Harvard Guide to Women's Health.* Cambridge, MA: Harvard University Press, 2004.
Rebecca A. Clark, Robert T. Maupin Jr., and Jill Hayes Hammer	*A Woman's Guide to Living with HIV Infection.* Baltimore: Johns Hopkins University Press, 2004.
George Creatsas, George Mastorakos, and George P. Chrousos, eds.	*Women's Health and Disease: Gynecologic and Reproductive Issues.* New York: New York Academy of Sciences, 2003.

178

Lynn P. Freedman   *Who's Got the Power? Transforming*
et al.   *Health Systems for Women and Chil-*
                   dren. Sterling, VA: Earthscan, 2005.

Marilyn Hughes   *Prime Time: The African American*
Gaston and Gayle   *Woman's Complete Guide to Midlife*
K. Porter   *Health and Wellness.* New York: One
                   World, 2003.

Adriana Gómez   *Reflections of Inequality: Women and*
and Deborah   *Mental Health.* Santiago, Chile: Latin
Meacham, eds.   American and Caribbean Women's
                   Health Network. 2001.

Diann S. Gregory   *Maternity and Women's Health.* Clif-
                   ton Park, NY: Delmar Learning,
                   2006.

Marcia C. Inhorn   *Infertility Around the Globe: New*
and Frank van   *Thinking on Childlessness, Gender,*
Balen, eds.   *and Reproductive Technologies,* Berke-
                   ley: University of California Press,
                   2002.

Institute of   *Exploring the Biological Contributions*
Medicine   *to Human Health: Does Sex Matter?*
                   Washington, DC: National Academy,
                   2001.

Miriam Jacobs   *Silent Invaders: Pesticides, Livelihoods*
and Barbara   *and Women's Health.* New York: Zed,
Dinham, eds.   2003.

Stanlie M. James   *Genital Cutting and Transnational*
and Claire C.   *Sisterhood: Disputing U.S. Polemics.*
Robertson, eds.   Urbana: University of Illinois Press,
                   2002.

Fran E. Kaiser, ed. *Women's Health Issues*. Philadelphia: W.B. Saunders, 2003.

Cheryl A. Kolander, Danny J. Ballard, and Cynthia K. Chandler — *Contemporary Women's Health: Issues for Today and the Future*. 2nd ed. Boston: McGraw-Hill, 2005.

Sana Loue and Martha Sajatovic, eds. — *Encyclopedia of Women's Health*. New York: Kluwer Academic/Plenum, 2004.

Robin M. Mathy and Shelly K. Kerr, eds. — *Lesbian and Bisexual Women's Mental Health*. Binghamton, NY: Haworth, 2003.

Susan McDonald and Christine Thompson, eds. — *Women's Health: A Handbook*. New York: Elsevier, 2005.

Mary Jane Minkin and Carol V. Wright — *A Woman's Guide to Menopause and Perimenopause*. New Haven: Yale University Press, 2005.

Elizabeth Ring-Cassidy and Ian Gentles — *Women's Health After Abortion: The Medical and Psychological Evidence*. 2nd ed. Toronto: DeVeber Institute for Bioethics and Social Research, 2003.

Jo Ann Rosenfeld, ed. — *Women's Health in Mid-life: A Primary Care Guide*. New York: Cambridge, 2004.

Kerri Durnell Schuiling and Frances E. Likis, eds. — *Women's Gynecologic Health*. Sudbury, MA: Jones and Bartlett, 2006.

Amy L. Sutton, ed.   *Women's Health Concerns Sourcebook.* 2nd ed. Detroit, MI: Omnigraphics, 2004.

Deborah Waller and Ann McPherson, ed.   *Women's Health.* 5th ed. New York: Oxford University Press, 2003.

Nanette Kass Wenger and Peter Collins, eds.   *Women and Heart Disease.* 2nd ed. New York: Taylor and Francis, 2005.

Nancy Fugate Woods and Margaret Heitkemper, eds.   *Women's Health.* Philadelphia: Saunders, 2004.

Periodicals

Laura Berman   "Women's Sexual Health Deserves Equal Attention," *USA Today,* November 23, 2004.

Christen Brownlee   "Monthly Cycle Changes Women's Brains," *Science News,* November 19, 2005.

Sandra Cortina   "Advancing Women's Health Care: Diagnostic, Treatment, and Social Factors of PMDD," *Women & Therapy,* 2005.

Tessa DeCarlo   "When Diets Turn Deadly," *Ladies' Home Journal,* June 2005.

Paula Dranov   "What Even Young Women Need to Know About Heart Disease," *Ladies' Home Journal,* February 2005.

Environmental Nutrition	"Health Concerns at Menopause: HRT Vs. Natural Remedies for Relief," January 2002.
FDA Consumer	"Moderate Physical Activity May Reduce Chronic Disease Risk in Older Women," March/April 2003.
Christine Gorman	"Menopause: Beyond Hot Flashes," *Time*, October 10, 2005.
Harvard Women's Health Watch	"Gender Matters: Heart Disease Risk in Women," May 2004.
Dana Hudepohl	"Living with Autoimmune Disease," *Woman's Day*, April 15, 2003.
JAMA: Journal of the American Medical Association	"Gender and Health," November 18, 2005.
Joanna Kerr	"State of Our Globe—Globalization & Women's Health," *Women & Environments International Magazine*, Fall 2003.
Gina Kolata	"Why Thin Is Fine, but Thinner Can Kill," *New York Times*, April 24, 2005.
Shiriki K. Kumanyika, Christiaan B. Morssink, and Marion Nestle	"Minority Women and Advocacy for Women's Health," *American Journal of Public Health*, September 2001.
Grace E. Park	"Women's Hearts," *Diabetes Forecast*, October 2005.

Tara Parker-Pope   "The Fear Factor: Women Continue to Shy Away from Hormone Therapy," *Wall Street Journal*, October 11, 2005.

Pharmaceutical Representative   "One in Four Non-elderly Women Forgoes Care Due to Costs," September 2005.

Prevention   "Unequal Treatment in the ER," July 2004.

Pulse   "Premenstrual Syndrome: Making Sense of the Options," February 8, 2005.

Lee Ann Runy   "Access to Insurance Impacts Women's Health Care," *Hospitals & Health Networks*, September 2005.

H. Wayne Sampson   "Alcohol and Other Factors Affecting Osteoporosis Risk in Women," *Alcohol Research & Health*, 2002.

Saturday Evening Post   "Women's Wellness," November/ December 2005.

Olive Shisana and Alicia Davids   "Correcting Gender Inequalities Is Central to Controlling HIV/AIDS," *Bulletin of the World Health Organization*, November 2004.

Anne Sutcliffe   "An Overview of Osteoporosis," *Nursing Standard*, September 21, 2005.

Marianne Szegedy-Maszak and Susan Brink   "It's All in Your Head, Honey," *U.S. News & World Report*, May 30, 2005.

Rosemarie Tong   "Towards a Feminist Global Bioethics: Addressing Women's Health Concerns Worldwide," *Health Care Analysis*, December 2001.

Moncef Zouali   "Taming Lupus," *Scientific American*, March 2005.

Index